A guide to research for podiatrists

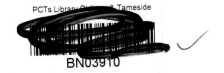

A guide to research for podiatrists

edited by Jackie Campbell

A guide to research for podiatrists
Jackie Campbell, ed.

ISBN: 978-1-905539-41-3

First published 2007

British Library Catalogue in Publication Data
A catalogue record for this book is available from the British Library.

Notice:
Clinical practice and medical knowledge constantly evolve. Standard safety precautions must be followed, but, as knowledge is broadened by research, changes in practice, treatment and drug therapy may become necessary or appropriate. Readers must check the most current product information provided by the manufacturer of each drug to be administered and verify the dosages and correct administration, as well as contraindications. It is the responsibility of the practitioner, utilising the experience and knowledge of the patient, to determine dosages and the best treatment for each individual patient. Neither the publisher nor the authors assume any liability for any injury and/or damage to persons or property arising from this publication.

The Publisher

To contact M&K Publishing write to:
M&K Update Ltd · The Old Bakery · St. John's Street
Keswick · Cumbria CA12 5AS

Tel: 01768 773030 · Fax: 01768 781099
Email: publishing@mkupdate.co.uk
www.mkupdate.co.uk

Designed & typeset in 11pt Usherwood Book by Mary Blood
Printed in England by

Contents

About the authors

Andrew Barnes is a clinically practising podiatrist working in Barnsley Primary Care Trust in Yorkshire. He is committed to developing the profession and has special interests in biomechanics and the development of evidence-based practice within podiatry. He was an active committee member of the Podiatric Research Forum for many years.

Dr Alan Borthwick is currently Lecturer at the School of Health Professions and Rehabilitation Sciences, University of Southampton. His work on the contemporary and historical sociology of the profession of podiatry is extensively published and he has presented his research in Europe, Australia, Canada and New Zealand.

Jackie Campbell is Professor of Neurophysiology at the University of Northampton, Research Coordinator for the Society of Chiropodists and Podiatrists, Chair of the Research Forum for Allied Health Professions and a freelance health research consultant. She is also a qualified statistician. She has wide-ranging research interests and experience but is particularly involved in pain research and research relating to the professions allied to medicine.

Dr Mike Curran is currently a Senior Lecturer working at the School of Health, University of Northampton. He has undertaken extensive research in the area of computers within podiatry and has published widely. His current research is on computational methods of gait and footprint recognition. He has recently completed a Medici Fellowship investigating how academic research may be commercialised and is currently undertaking an MBA.

Dr Lisa Farndon is a Podiatric Development Facilitator for the Podiatry Service, Sheffield Primary Care Trust, where she is involved in service development, research and audit. She has been working as an NHS podiatrist for the past 20 years and her main research interests are professional development, patient empowerment and qualitative research methods.

A guide to research for podiatrists

Dr Farina Hashmi is a Senior Lecturer and Research Coordinator at the Division of Podiatry, School of Health Professions, University of Brighton. Her research interests include dermatology, wound biochemistry and tissue mechanics. Farina has published in international academic journals and has contributed to national and international conferences. She is a reviewer for several academic journals and grant-funding bodies. She is also a member of the Research and Development Committee for the Society of Chiropodists and Podiatrists, UK.

Professor Kate Springett is Head of the Department of Allied Health Professions, Canterbury Christ Church University College. Her research and clinical areas of expertise and interest include tissue viability, diabetes and dermatology, skin and musculoskeletal ultrasound imaging and low level laser therapy within an interprofessional rehabilitation context.

Professor Wesley Vernon is Head of Sheffield Podiatry Service, Research Lead for Sheffield Primary Care Trust and a Visiting Professor at Staffordshire University. His predominant research interests are forensic podiatry and workforce and developmental aspects of podiatry, and he has gained national and international recognition for achievements in these fields.

A guide to research for podiatrists

Preface

Evidence-based practice is now expected of all healthcare professionals. It is becoming even more vital with the advent of practice-based commissioning for those within the NHS who need to respond to increasingly well-informed and discerning patients within both private and public sectors. There is now also a much greater emphasis on continuing professional development (CPD) with the requirement that all allied health professionals (AHPs) must regularly demonstrate their engagement with CPD and reflect on how it has improved their practice in order to continue their registration with the Health Professions Council.

Within podiatry, there is therefore an expectation that, at the very least, all podiatrists should be users of research. We should all be able to read about research-based evidence for practice and apply it to our own situation in order to help our profession progress. At the same time, more podiatrists need to contribute actively to this evidence by undertaking research studies themselves to collect new information.

Podiatry Research is an edited collection of articles on the process of research in podiatry. Previously published as monthly instalments in the journal *Podiatry Now*, between October 2006 and September 2007, each one has now been updated and edited for this book. The collection is designed for those who are new to research, or who just need a reminder of the principles. It is intended to give a general introduction to each of the topics rather than equip the reader with all the skills needed to carry it out.

This overview should be useful to those who need to find, read and understand research evidence to incorporate into their own practice, and as a first port of call for those planning on collecting their own research evidence. It also forms a source of self-directed study material that can be reflected on in a CPD portfolio or used as a general handbook for podiatry students who are studying research methods as part of their undergraduate course.

The topics covered include: defining a research question, finding existing evidence, research design, data collection, research funding, ethical approval, data analysis, dissemination of results and putting your findings into practice – for both quantitative and qualitative research.

Chapter 1
The why, who and what of podiatry research

Wesley Vernon and Jackie Campbell

The recent development of the podiatry profession

It is constantly suggested that, as podiatrists, we need to research, but what does this really mean? This question can be particularly problematic in a profession such as podiatry, where there has not been a strong research basis for practice in the past.

Until relatively recently, podiatrists were trained by simply being presented with what was considered to be the knowledge required to be able to practise. At the time, very few podiatrists considered that chiropody, as the profession was then generally called, would change and develop, to become the profession it now is, with a much wider scope of practice requiring a somewhat stronger foundation.

The change to a degree-based profession was fundamental to many of the developments which have taken place. Degree status brought with it the world of the reflective practitioner – one in which podiatrists began to consider carefully what it was they were doing in their practice, whether it could be improved, why they practised in a particular manner, whether it could be justified and whether there might be an entirely different way of going about the task in hand. Information was no longer accepted at face value, but instead was scrutinised, criticised, questioned and used to raise other questions. In other words, podiatrists were being prepared to understand, use and undertake their own research.

Although this was uncomfortable, it could be suggested that this change came about at just the right time. Things were beginning to change as never before, particularly in the business of healthcare and its delivery.

A guide to research for podiatrists

Healthcare policy changes

**Policy
changes**

Policy changes affecting the NHS particularly reflect this different scenario. It is no longer acceptable to do something on the basis of custom and practice alone. Within the NHS, the government has both stated explicitly and implied, through various modernisation policies and their supporting documentation, that all healthcare must improve. Traditional ways of working are being challenged all the time, especially in terms of efficiency and effectiveness [1–5]. At the same time, there are considerations of safety and risk to be taken on board and concepts of patient satisfaction and service quality to be developed and understood. In other words, clinical governance frameworks need to be implemented and developed further.

Evidence-based practice

**Evidence-based
practice**

Many of the intentions stated in the new health policies have implied that new initiatives are required, based on a sound understanding of what is effective clinically. Modern professional groups are now expected to make clinical, managerial and policy decisions, based on sound information derived through research findings and other scientific developments – in other words a knowledge-based health service is being created.

Such improvements in understanding need to be based on research. High-quality care, best practice initiatives and the development of improved services need to be worked through rigorously. This means that practice should be researched and then modified, based on the findings of that research. It should be evidence-based. These changes have in turn led to the creation of bodies such as the National Institute for Health and Clinical Excellence (NICE) – the national body responsible for providing guidance on the promotion of good health and the prevention and treatment of ill health (www.nice.org.uk). NICE bases its recommendations on the best available evidence, gathered through research.

The suggestion is that best practice in healthcare will need to be demonstrated and underpinned by research. Without research, a professional group will not only be in danger of being seen as a second-class service, but could also be seen as unable to justify its own existence in terms of clinical effectiveness and could in turn become 'obsolete'.

These required changes are not, however, restricted to the NHS working environment and need to be considered in all areas of practice. Podiatry is now regulated by the Health Professions Council and this regulation demands fitness for practice amongst its regulated registrants (www.hpc-uk.org). The test of whether or not practice has been provided to an acceptable level is that of the reasonable practitioner and, in this sense, a podiatrist's standard of practice will be judged against that which can be considered reasonable, or typical. Improvements in practice within large public service providers such as the NHS will necessarily therefore shift standards and expectations upwards across all sectors of provision and this in turn suggests that all practising podiatrists will rely on research-derived understanding to justify what they do clinically.

Why is research needed for the development of podiatry?

Why research?

The case can therefore be made for the need for the podiatry profession to develop and improve on the grounds that there are multiple and strong policy requirements to modernise practice, with a particular emphasis on evidence-based approaches and to improve approaches to clinical governance. Why then is research needed in relation to these requirements?

Research can be defined as 'systematic investigation to establish facts or principles or to collect information on a subject' or 'investigations into a subject, problem etc' [6]. The term research in itself, however, can be seen as being incomplete. The complete and accurate term should arguably be 'research and development'. This has been defined as 'activity concerned with applying the results of scientific research to develop new products and improve existing ones' [6]. This definition, with its emphasis on application, helps explain why research is needed in order to underpin clinical practice.

Research according to tried and tested definitions is fundamental and integral to the process of development and improvement. If there is to be development and improvement of any type, then research will be required. Research provides the best means of describing and understanding a given situation through the rigour required in research activities. Simple rhetoric or anecdotally based arguments are no longer adequate when attempting to justify a direction for change, especially when many of the medical and other health-related disciplines are presenting research-based information to justify their own positions. Development without research may therefore no longer be adequate. An evidence base needs to be presented in order for new developments to be accepted.

There are additional problems in attempting to develop the profession without research. If developments take place without coordinated, publicised research, there is a danger of constantly re-inventing the wheel, slowing down improvements within the profession and leading to wasted activity amongst the busy practitioners involved. Developments without research can also lead to errors and the potential for the profession to go down 'blind alleys' in the search for improvement. Through both the stringency and outputs (presentations, publications and so on) required in the research process, the possibility of such problems occurring is reduced.

Who should take part in research?

Who should take part?

If we accept the need for research, who should carry it out? It has previously been suggested that there should be some level of involvement throughout the profession [7], although not everyone will need to become active researchers. At the most basic level, there is an argument to suggest that everyone does need to be research-sensitive, with an awareness of the value of research, how to critique published research for themselves and how to adjust their practice continually in order to take such research findings into consideration. In this way, podiatric education will develop and best practice be followed at all times. Such awareness would ideally extend beyond purely clinical aspects of podiatry and take into account research in other areas including, for instance, organisational development.

The why, who and what of podiatry research

At the next level, a core of 'research-able' podiatrists will be needed in order to produce the research upon which future development will depend. These individuals are likely to be career researchers in the new health structures, working within roles currently being proposed [8]. Obviously fewer research-able than research-sensitive professionals will be required, and research will be restricted to those who wish to develop the necessary skills.

Finally, an even smaller number of research leaders are needed to drive a research vision for the profession. These leaders will have the interest, motivation and ambition to lead the profession in the required directions. They will also need a previous track record of research to provide an in-depth understanding of research, its practice and value. Such leadership would not, however, work without the broader involvement of the entire profession.

What does research involve?

What is involved?

The research process is similar to many developmental activities. It requires a good idea or question to investigate, a strategy that can be used to collect and analyse the information to illuminate the idea or question, and a method of disseminating the findings to others. The steps to be taken, and the methods used, are very similar for research, audit and evaluation. The main difference is that research should be generalisable to a wider population, whereas audit and evaluation tend to be undertaken locally. Additionally, the questions for audit are usually predetermined, and involve comparison of local results with a predetermined standard. However, research skills are involved in all these activities.

Figure 1.1 is adapted from a publication produced by the NHS Executive [9] and summarises the steps that make up a typical research project. The subsequent chapters in this book will expand on these stages.

A guide to research for podiatrists

Figure 1.1

Summary of the steps that make up a typical research project

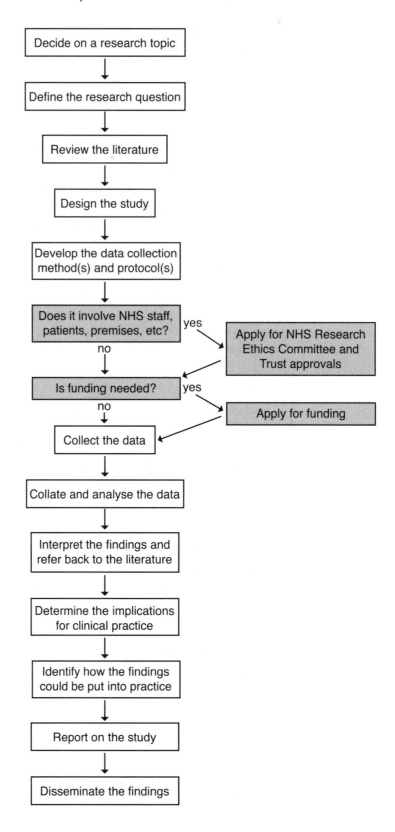

References

[1] Department of Health. *A Health Service of All Talents: Developing the NHS workforce.* Consultation document on the review of workforce planning (London: DH, 2000).

[2] Department of Health. *Meeting the Challenge: A strategy for the allied health professions* (London: DH, 2000).

[3] Department of Health. *Agenda for Change* (London: DH, 2003).

[4] Department of Health. *Commissioning a Patient-led NHS* (London: DH, 2005).

[5] Department of Health. *The NHS Plan: A plan for investment, a plan for reform* (London: DH, 2000).

[6] J. Sinclair (ed.) *Collins English Dictionary* (Glasgow: Harper Collins, 1995).

[7] W. Vernon. Research in Podiatry: Why do we need it, what do we need to do and what does it mean for me? *Podiatry Now* 5 (2002), 466.

[8] Department of Health. *Best Research for Best Health* (London: DH, 2006).

[9] NHS Executive. Designing a research study. In *Achieving Effective Practice: a clinical effectiveness and research information pack for nurses, midwives and health visitors* (London: DH, 1998).

Chapter 2
Defining the research question

Kate Springett and Jackie Campbell

Getting your research question right is absolutely crucial to the rest of the research process. Getting the right answer to the wrong question is clearly going to waste an awful lot of time and resources. But the main problem is not so much asking the wrong question as not properly defining the right question.

This chapter will assume that you have identified a general area that you are interested in researching and give guidance as to how to take that idea and shape it into a researchable question. This process should be the same whether you are searching existing literature for the answer or preparing to design and conduct your own research study. It is neither simple nor quick. It can take days, weeks or sometimes months – depending upon the complexity of the problem – to arrive at a clear, concise and accurate question. It is not worth rushing; time spent now will save irritation and frustration later.

What is a research question?

When you have a problem to solve, a question for which an answer is needed, then you have to do some work to find that answer. Sometimes this information is available in the literature; sometimes you need to start from scratch because little or no information exists. Either way you need to spend time deciding what the problem is, what the nature of the problem is, and what it is that you really want to find out in relation to it.

Turning this research project into a non-biased and precise question – a research question – helps you understand how to answer it. If you are doing a review of the literature, you need a research question; if you want to find out about the efficacy of an intervention through a clinical study, you need a research question; if you want to explore patients' perceptions of a management approach, you need a research question. Whether your planned work is likely to use a qualitative or quantitative approach, you need a research question. A research question also acts as an *aide mémoire*. It helps you keep focused on your area of enquiry. This is particularly helpful if you find that you get side-tracked easily when you search the literature.

Focusing your question

Focusing your question

The key to defining a research question is focus. The end product needs to be a specific query that is explicit in what it is looking for. The process of defining the question is therefore essentially one of taking a broad topic area and narrowing it down until you have a question that can be answered fully. How much focus is required depends to some extent on how much research you are intending to do to answer it. Given unlimited time and resources, a question such as 'What is the best management regime for metatarsalgia?' might be answerable, but it would take a long time to research all possible treatments, for all possible populations of patients. In doing so, you would probably break the question down into bite-sized chunks such as 'How effective is a conservative approach compared with surgical intervention for the most common cause of metatarsalgia in adults?'. These chunks are effectively just better-defined research questions.

Once you have decided upon the research question, you can then choose which research approach (qualitative, quantitative or both) is most appropriate. The research question governs everything else in the research process – the methodology, the data collection, the data analysis and, of course, the findings. This is why it is such a vital first step.

Booth and Fry-Smith [1] also suggest that additional components included in the process of focusing the question may include:

- the study designs you are interested in (e.g. randomised controlled trials);
- the context in which relevant studies have been undertaken, or whether there are factors that will limit its applicability to the question being asked;

- language restrictions (e.g. English only – note potential for language bias);
- any date restrictions on the period the literature review will cover (e.g. if updating an existing review).

The PICO approach

The PICO approach

One approach to limiting the scope of the topic area is to use the PICO framework. Although this approach was developed around evidence-based medicine [2] and was therefore designed for clinical studies, it can be adapted to any research context. An adapted version is used here. The main elements of the research question can be broken down into four areas:

P: Patient, population or problem

What are the characteristics of the patient or population?

What is the condition or disease you are interested in?

I: Intervention or exposure

What do you want to do with this patient/population (e.g. treat, diagnose, observe)?

C: Comparison

What is the alternative to the intervention (e.g. placebo, different drug, surgery)?

O: Outcome

What are the relevant outcomes (e.g. morbidity, death, complications)?

Figure 2.1 (overleaf) is a step-by-step guide (adapted from [2]) to help you refine, define and focus the problem you have come across and need to solve and to turn it into a research question .

The following section explains how to use this framework to define your research question. Allow time for this development. Some worked examples are given at the end of this section.

P – Patient, population or problem

Starting at the beginning, with the first two boxes on the flowchart related to 'P', write your thoughts down: capture them on paper to control them. What is the nature of the problem that you have come across and need an answer for?

For a complex area, or one you cannot see your way through, you may find highlighting different written thoughts in different colours helps. Some people use spider diagrams (mind maps) to

A guide to research for podiatrists

Figure 2.1

Using the PICO approach to defining a research question

Using the PICO approach to defining a research question

 P What is the problem that you have come across in practice and need an answer for? What is the patient group that is relevant to the area you need to look into?

Tease this information out; break it into sub-units. What are you interested in? Pick out key words and phrases that capture this and turn into questions.

 I What do you need to do with your patients/population, or involve yourself with, to find out the nature of, or answer to, the problem? What information do you want to capture? What intervention do you want to investigate? What is it that you want to assess and diagnose or evaluate? What is it that you want to observe?

Keep asking yourself questions to help you identify and refine what it is that you want to find out. Include the points you arrive at in your prototype RQ.

 C Are there comparisons to be made, or differences to establish? Is monitoring all that is needed? Do you expect themes or groups of characteristics to emerge, e.g. from observation? This section may not be relevant to your plans.

Your prototype RQ needs to reflect what you need and plan to do. Has your RQ captured all components so far?

O What outcome(s) is/are relevant? What is it that you will be measuring, observing, assessing?

Try writing out your question. After a few days, does it seem to you to be the right question? Tell others your qustion. Do they understand what you want to get at? If not, re-word and refine.

Using comments and returning to your problem, have you covered all the points you need in your prototype RQ? If not, re-word and further refine.

Does the RQ indicate precisely the required components without bias?
Yes – you have defined your RQ.

P = patient, population, problem; **I** = intervention or exposure;
C = comparison; **O** = outcome; **RQ** = research question)
Source: Adapted from [2]

show links; others like cutting and pasting to show links. Once you have your initial thoughts down on paper, discard the ones that seem irrelevant to the problem and link others together. What are the main points, the key components or the sub-units that strike you? Try turning these into questions.

Leave what you have written for a few days, return to it with a fresh eye and discard those elements that seem wrong or do not really seem to fit with what you want to find out. Using the remaining outline question(s), find out whether other people understand what you want to enquire about. If not it is 'back to the drawing board'.

I – Intervention or exposure

Moving onto the two ovals relating to 'I', begin to look at including in your prototype research question what it is you need to do to find out what you want to find out. Use the reading you have done around this area to help specify what this is.

You may want to look at treatments for a particular condition, in which case you will need to state the intervention, treatment or management approach in your prototype RQ. If you plan to evaluate patient data, there may be an audit process (such as an annual review) that you plan to use and this needs to be included within your RQ. If you want to explore patients' commentaries, your approach may be through interview or a focus group and this also needs to be reflected within your RQ. Whatever it is that you intend, include this in your question.

C – Comparison

This stage asks you to consider whether there are additional things that you want or need to include. Do you want to compare treatments? If so, you will need to include the first treatment within your prototype research question along with the treatment you plan as a comparison.

If there are no direct comparisons to be made, you will still need to include within your RQ that you, for example, plan to monitor uptake of services over time. It may be that you plan to explore patients' perceptions concerning their health but need to do this in different contexts or times of disorder onset. This information needs to be included within your question.

However, it may be that this comparison is not relevant at all to your study, in which case leave it out!

O – Outcome

This stage encourages you to include in your RQ what the outcome is that you will be measuring or exploring. If centred around a clinical study you may be interested in outcomes including time (e.g. time to healing), whether the condition has resolved, costs of the interventions, patients' perceptions of the benefit of the intervention and so on.

Now you have included all the parts of your RQ, it is time to leave what you have composed again for at least two days. Returning with a fresh eye, does your RQ say what you wanted it to say? Try it out with colleagues. Do they understand what you intend? If not, re-word and refine and then you will arrive at your well-built research question.

Some worked examples

Some examples

Example 1

General nature/area of problem: We use phenol for nail matrix ablation. Is this really the best way and the best substance to use?

Population	people with ingrowing toe nails
Intervention	total or partial nail ablation using NaOH
Comparison	total or partial nail ablation using phenol
Outcome	post-operative pain, regrowth, healing rate, satisfaction

RQ: Is sodium hydroxide a viable alternative to phenol for nail matrix ablation?

Example 2

General nature/area of problem: With the National Service Framework for Older People, we need to find a way of targeting our 'at risk' population. How can we do this?

Population	people aged 75 years and over
Intervention	annual foot health monitoring
Comparison	no monitoring
Outcome	effectiveness of health check tool for diagnosis of high-risk podiatric conditions and no professional foot care

RQ: Can an annual foot health check for the over-75s detect high-risk conditions that would otherwise be missed?

Example 3

General nature/area of problem: Outcome measures tend not to capture the impact of rheumatoid arthritis (RA) on patients' daily lives in a way that has a patient focus, but there is limited information in the literature about what it is that worries people with RA as far as their feet are concerned. How can we find this out?

Population	people with RA
Problem	nature of concerns
Intervention	interview, focus group
Comparison	no comparison; themes describing nature of concerns expected to develop
Outcome	identification of a range of issues, e.g. anxiety, uncertainty, frustration

RQ: What concerns do people with RA have, relating to their feet and mobility?

Conclusion

Following a structured process in developing your research question means that you do not miss out stages of thinking. After a while this step-by-step method becomes second nature and you will not know that you are going through these stages. Nevertheless, you will still need to allow time for this stage of the research process. It is an important one: a focused research question is essential to the success of the research which follows.

References

[1] A. Booth and A. Fry-Smith. Developing the research question. In *Etext on Health Technology Assessment (HTA) Information Resources*, ed. L-A. Topfer and I. Auston. Available at www.nlm.nih.gov. Accessed 2.7.07.

[2] W. Richardson and M. Wilson. On questions, background and foreground. *Evidence Based Healthcare Newsletter*, 17 (1997), 8–9.

Chapter 3
Finding the literature for research projects

Farina Hashmi

During our day-to-day clinical work we make observations that cause us to question why we practise in the way we do. This type of questioning encourages us to search the existing body of literature for answers. When we do, it sometimes become apparent that there are gaps in the existing knowledge that need to be addressed and this, in essence, forms the basis of a research question and subsequently a research project.

There is an abundance of clinical research publications: some represent high-quality research; some are poorly written. With this variability in mind it is imperative to carry out a careful and thorough search of the literature, armed with the necessary skill to analyse the standards of the publications critically. This skill is something that you need to develop and should be a prerequisite for any type of clinical research.

Finding good-quality healthcare information on the internet

Internet information

Healthcare information on the internet should be viewed with a critical eye, as much of it represents poor-quality evidence. The internet resource INTUTE (formerly known as BIOME) (www.intute.ac.uk) publishes some useful guidelines on evaluating websites. The basic questions to ask when looking at a web page are:

● When was the page last updated?

● Who is responsible for the contents?

● Are references quoted in full?

A guide to research for podiatrists

Academic journals

Academic journals

Journals are used for publishing results of academic research and are subject to peer review prior to publication, ensuring that the quality of any paper meets a specific standard. At the time of publication an article could be only 6 to 18 months old, giving journals a clear advantage over books, which take longer to be published. There are over 25,000 peer-reviewed journals and many more that are not peer reviewed, the majority of which are available online. Libraries will subscribe to services which give free access to many journals but you may have to pay to download an article if the journal is not included in the library's subscription, or if you are not a member of such a library.

Bibliographic databases

Bibligraphic databases

Bibliographic databases provide searchable lists of individual journal articles and allow the user to find articles on a given subject by typing in words that describe that subject. Databases provide citations of articles (author, title, source, date, volume and page numbers) and often provide abstracts (brief summaries of the article content) and links to the full-text article.

There is an ever-increasing number of online medical databases hosting peer-reviewed academic journals. Each database provides a description of the types of journals archived (see Table 3.1 below). The two most popular, large, searchable online databases for clinical research journals are Medline (a component of Pubmed) and Science Direct. Their popularity stems from their broad subject coverage and the publications that they hold which report original research.

Table 3.1

Useful online medical databases of academic journals

Useful online medical databases of academic journals

Database name	Core subjects
Abstracts in New Technology and Engineering (ANTE)	*Biotechnology, medical technology and engineering*
Allied and Complementary Medicine (AMED)	*Complementary medicine, physiotherapy, occupational therapy, podiatry, palliative care*

Finding the literature for research projects

Applied Social Sciences Index and Abstracts (ASSIA)	*Health, psychology, sociology, economics, education, human resource management*
Australian Education Index (AEI)	*Curriculum, education policy planning and administration, vocational education and training, evaluation and assessment, educational psychology and sociology*
British Education Index	*Curriculum, education policy planning and administration, vocational education and training, evaluation and assessment, educational psychology and sociology*
British Nursing Index	*Nursing, midwifery, evidence-based practice, disabilities, reflective practice*
Cochrane Library	*Systematic reviews, Cochrane Central Register for Controlled Trials, Cochrane Database of Methodology Reviews, Health Technology Assessment Database, NHS Economic Evaluation Database*
Cumulative Index to Nursing and Allied Health Literature (CINAHL)	*Health education, physiotherapy and social services in healthcare*
Emerald Fulltext	*Management, human resource management*
Expanded Academic ASAP	*Science and technology and social sciences*
Index to Theses	*Higher degrees at universities in the UK*
IngentaConnect	*General*
ISI Journal Citation Reports	*A comprehensive source for journal evaluation, using citation data drawn from scholarly and technical journals worldwide. Coverage is multidisciplinary and international.*
ISI Proceedings – Science and Technology Edition	*Published literature of conferences, symposia, seminars, workshops and conventions in a wide range of disciplines in science and technology*
ISI Web of Science	*Science Citation Index, Social Sciences Citation Index and Arts and Humanities Citation Index*
PsycINFO	*Psychology and psychological aspects of related disciplines such as medicine, nursing, sociology, education, pharmacology and physiology*
Wiley Interscience (Journals published by Wiley)	*(Over 400 journals.) Science, education, psychology*
Zetoc (The British Library's Electronic Table of Contents Service)	*(20,000 journals and 16,000 conference proceedings) General*

A guide to research for podiatrists

Careful thought needs to be given to the way that these databases are searched to produce papers on the topic that you are interested in. Databases may use different methods of searching and the advice of a librarian is often invaluable at this stage. A well-defined research question is also essential.

It is worth investing time in working through a comprehensive search strategy and keeping a record of what search terms you used. You will find that the search strategy has to be refined. If the search results in thousands of papers then it needs to be focused more closely on the area of interest; if too few papers are found then the search terms may need to be expanded. Also, you may find that the keywords you are searching on are ambiguous and produce papers on entirely unconnected topics.

There are strategies that can be used such as excluding search terms, using 'wild cards', defining sub-areas, defining study populations or publication dates. Again, the help of a librarian can be useful here. The main advantage of saving the search history is that you can repeat a well-crafted search strategy easily, without having to start from scratch. You can also be assured that the same thorough search is being carried out each time a search is conducted. A description of the search strategy is often required in publications.

Useful online search tips

The following tips may be useful:

- If the relevant details of the paper are to hand (for example, the title of the article, the authors and the year of publication) the search for a specific article is relatively straightforward. Select the type of search you wish to carry out (for example, by author) and type the details into the search engine. In the case of searching by author, a list of publications may appear. The more details you have, the greater the chance of minimising the number of citations.
- If you do not know which article you need (a situation which is often the case in the early stages of developing a research question), the literature search requires a more strategic approach. The most common methods involve the use of keywords.
  - The use of Boolean logic adds to the efficiency and accuracy of the search by allowing for the keywords used to be combined in a logical and standard way. This involves

incorporating terms such as AND, NOT and OR (relational operators) into the search.

– A thesaurus is available in many databases. It adds more scope to the search by suggesting words or phases that are similar to those you are using.

Other productive ways of gaining the desired information in the field of interest are 'snowball' methods such as seeking key references from other papers, electronic citation tracking and measures as simple as browsing library shelves and discussing literature with colleagues [1].

Critical appraisal

Critical appraisal

When reading a research paper, it is essential to adopt a critical approach. The critiquing process ranges from simply noting the layout of the report to challenging the content of the paper. There are specific factors to consider when appraising each section of a research paper:

- The title should reflect the content of the article.
- The abstract is a brief synopsis of the complete paper. It should describe what was investigated, what methods were used and the rationale for selecting these methods. It should finish by describing what was found and what conclusions, if any, were drawn from the findings.
- A good introduction will contain a background to the study explaining to the reader the importance of the study. It must have a review of the relevant literature, including some theoretical support for the study. This should ultimately lead to a statement of the research question and the hypotheses tested.
- The methods section must accurately and concisely describe what was done to answer the research question and test the hypotheses. The sample selection (highlighting the inclusion and exclusion criteria), the equipment used and the procedures carried out must be explicit in the report. A well-written methods section should make it possible for the reader to replicate the study.
- The results should report what the investigators found. The data must be clear and easy to understand, using appropriate tables

and graphs. The correct statistical tests should be used to test the hypothesis or research question.

● The discussion should be informed by previous research in the field of interest. In this section, clear statements should be made about whether the hypotheses set out in the introduction have been confirmed or refuted by the results of the study. It is at this point that the limitations of the study are acknowledged. It is always good practice to summarise the findings describing what has been found by this piece of research.

Table 3.2 (below) gives examples of the sort of questions that could be considered when critically appraising a paper.

Table 3.2

A list of the key questions for critical appraisal of a research paper

Key questions for critical appraisal of a research paper

Introduction	Does the study ask a clear, focused question? How relevant is the problem? Does the research challenge or add to existing ideas?
Method	Is the choice of method suitable to the problem? Does it answer the research question? Does it test the hypothesis? Has the study been conducted with sufficient objectivity and control? Are the size and the composition of the samples representative of the groups of interest? Does the study have enough participants to to be significant? How valid and reliable are the instruments? If new instruments are used, how have they been piloted?
Results	How are the results presented? What is the main result? How precise are the results? Are all important outcomes considered so that the results can be applied? If the results are statistically significant, what is the clinical significance, if any?
Discussion	What are the limitations of the study? How could the work have been improved? How valid and reliable are the results? Can the findings be generalised? What are the indications of the research? What are the implications for clinical practice? Are alternative interpretations possible? Are the conclusions drawn from the data logical or do they go beyond the data? Is the report sufficiently critical of the methods employed? Does the study provide acceptable recommendations for practice?

Finding the literature for research projects

Summary

Once a research question has been identified, it needs to be supported or challenged by the evidence in the field. In the absence of this information it is difficult to decide on the direction in which the research should go.

In order to feel confident that the topic of research is one that may add to the existing knowledge in the field, you must be confident that all possible sources of literature have been investigated. This is achieved by a structured approach to searching the literature and constantly revisiting the literature throughout the research process.

References

[1] T. Greenhalgh and R. Peacock. Effectiveness and Efficiency of Search Methods in Systematic Reviews of Complex Evidence: Audit of primary sources. *British Medical Journal* 331 (2005), 1064–5.

Further reading

J. Bell. *Doing Your Research Project. A guide for first time researchers in education, health and social science,* 4th edn (Maidenhead: Open University Press, 2005).

G. M. Hall. *How to Write a Paper*, 3rd edn (London: BMJ Publishing Group, 2003).

C. Partridge and R. Barnitt. *Research Guidelines: A handbook for therapists* (London: Heinemann Medical Books, 1986).

Chapter 4
Finding new evidence – research design
Alan Borthwick, Lisa Farndon and Jackie Campbell

Conventionally, designs for research studies are divided into two categories: quantitative and qualitative. The choice of design should follow from your research question to ensure that data is collected and analysed in a way that will answer that question. However, the form that the research question takes is largely a function of underlying philosophy and the motivation for the research in the first place.

This chapter examines the main types of philosophical research stances as these underpin the resulting research methodologies. The main characteristics of quantitative and qualitative designs are outlined and, finally, some of the most common ways of carrying out research are described.

Research philosophies

Research philosophies

The main models of enquiry used in academic research are the positivist and the interpretative models.

The positivist model:
- is the natural science model
- is based on testing theories and hypotheses
- insists on objectivity and neutrality, avoiding personal bias
- requires that the researcher controls the theoretical framework, sampling frames and the structure of the research
- involves developing theory and concepts before data collection – seeks to falsify the initial hypothesis
- favours quantitative methods.

The interpretative model:
- has its roots in philosophy, history and anthropology
- centres on interpretation and creation of meaning by human beings

- accepts subjective reality
- looks at understanding rather than explanation
- regards context as crucial
- requires that researchers are reflexive, not objective
- favours qualitative methods.

Quantitative versus qualitative designs

Quantitative v. qualitative designs

The search for new knowledge can be approached in many ways. The approach taken depends on the nature and type of the research problem and the philosophical stance of the researcher (amongst other things). The most important factor, however, is that the methods should be chosen that will answer the research question.

There is also a link between research design and analytical methods. Future chapters in this series will focus on quantitative and qualitative data analysis but it is worth noting that this terminology can be confusing. For example, quantitative data is measurable data that can be represented by a number but it can be collected using a qualitative methodology. (For instance, you may want to collect data about the age range of your interviewees.) Similarly, qualitative data can be collected using quantitative methods. (For instance, you might invite unstructured comments as part of a questionnaire.)

Table 4.1 (below) compares the main features of quantitative and qualitative research designs.

Table 4.1

Main features of qualitative and qualitative research designs

	Qualitative design	Quantitative design
Aim	• Not generalisable • Exploration of participants' meaning • Understanding, generation of theory from data	• Generalisable results • Search for causal explanations • Testing hypotheses, prediction, control
Approach	• Broad focus, process-orientated • Context-bound, mostly natural setting • Getting close to the data	• Narrow focus, product-orientated • Context-free, often in artificial setting

Finding new evidence – research design

Sample	• Participants, informants • Flexible sampling which develops during research • Small samples, may be random, purposive, opportunistic	• Respondents, subjects, participants • Sample frame fixed before research starts • Usually need large samples, randomised
Data collection	• In-depth non-standardised interviews • Participant observation • Documents, photographs, videos, etc	• Questionnaire • Standardised interviews • Structured observation • Controlled trials, etc
Analysis	• Thematic, latent content analysis • Grounded theory, ethnographic analysis, etc	• Statistical analysis • Graphs, descriptions, etc
Validity	• Trustworthiness • Authenticity	• Validity • Reliability
Outcome	• A story • An ethnography • A theory	• Measurable results • Evidence to disprove a null hypothesis
Relationships	• Direct involvement of researcher • Research relationship close	• Limited involvement of researcher • Research relationship distant

Whilst this table presents qualitative and quantitative methodologies as two halves of a dichotomy, in reality there is a continuum of approaches between the two extremes with some blurring in the middle. Structured interviews are an example of this. Although it is generally accepted that interviews are a qualitative research method, asking short questions which do not invite wide-ranging responses from a highly structured and standardised interview schedule could be viewed as a positivist approach and has many of the attributes of quantitative research.

Some specific research designs within these two broad approaches are described below.

Qualitative research designs

Qualitative designs

Qualitative research designs are generally built around three main data collection methods: interviews, observations and documents. Each of these categories consists of a range of design types and features. The choice is dependent on the research question. Most qualitative studies will have exploratory, descriptive and explanatory elements, in order to establish what is happening in an area of enquiry and be able to understand and explain it. It will frequently involve the generation of a theory, framework or model from the data collected. It does not usually involve controlling events or manipulating variables (for example, making an intervention to change something).

Categorisation of qualitative research design is often based on the theoretical underpinning of a particular research question. For example, examining the culture of a group of people is classified as ethnography, investigating the lived experience is classified as phenomenology and developing theories which are grounded in reality is classified as grounded theory.

A case study design is used here as an exemplar of the practical aspects of qualitative research design. It may involve a mix of quantitative and qualitative methods, such as interviews and questionnaires, or it may involve a mix of purely qualitative measures, such as interviews and documentary analysis. For the purposes of this chapter, we will confine the case study approach to purely qualitative methods, of which there may be several. These are summarised below according to the main data collection methods used.

Interviews

Interviews

The interview is a long-established method of collecting research data and one that involves talking with research participants. Selection of this method is dependent on what the underlying research question is seeking to uncover – who would best know the answers. Time or financial constraints can influence the form of the interview, as well as the question being posed or the number of participants involved.

Interviews may take a range of different forms with different purposes: from key actor interviews to focus group interviews to telephone interviews. They may be standardised, involving pre-determined lists of short questions invoking short answers, or exploratory, involving an open, free-style, fluid agenda. Each of these is selected for a particular, specific reason and the research design is often concerned with getting in-depth information and meaning from relatively few participants.

For example, if the research question sought to understand the reasons why the Society of Chiropodists and Podiatrists (SCP) withdrew from membership of the Federation International des Podologues (FIP), as it did in 1975, and why it chose to rejoin in 1978 [1], the design would probably involve both interview and documentary sources of data collection. Interviews might take several different forms, depending on the sample of respondents being sought. For instance, you could obtain the perspectives of branch members, who constitute the grass roots of the organisation, possibly by face-to-face semi-structured interviews, which would allow the researcher to ask a pre-set list of questions whilst being able to elaborate with further questions if new issues arose during the course of the interview.

However, to truly understand the reasons for the decision, you would need to interview the people who made the decision, who would be the members of the SCP's Council, who lead the organisation and make the policy decisions. These would be the key actors – those with a particular knowledge of the events being studied, usually with direct involvement in it, and who need to be selected for this specialist knowledge, rather than randomly sampled. The point is that, although branch members may have views on the reasons for withdrawing from and rejoining the FIP, the SCP Council members, having taken the decision, would be the respondents best able to provide the answers.

It might be (hypothetically) possible to hold a focus group interview with those Council members most involved in the decision. This would allow data to be collected in one interview, and therefore avoid having to negotiate access to individuals separately. It also provides an opportunity to capture the dynamic of the meeting and the interactions between members. As these events took place some years ago, there may be fewer key actors available to speak with, in which case documentary sources would become even more important. These factors would inform the research design, which might change as the study progresses. As you can see, it is not always necessary, or desirable, to interview large numbers of people in order to enhance the validity of the findings, nor to seek generalisability. In this particular case, the aim is to access a small number of specially targeted individuals.

Telephone interviews can also be used, particularly when access to the interviewees is difficult because of geographical distance (if the person you want to speak with lives in Australia for instance), or perhaps because the respondents prefer to conduct the interview that way. Nowadays it is also possible to conduct online interviews, using email or other forms of electronic communication [2, 3].

In each case, the research question, and the practicalities associated with it, will determine the overall design of the study and the specific methods used.

Documentary sources

Documentary sources

Documents can consist of almost any type of record of events – from journal articles and editorials, adverts, newspaper articles, video clips, photographs and emails to minutes of meetings, personal letters, memoranda, personal diaries, and even gravestone inscriptions [4]. Documents do not need to be published to be legitimately used as data sources. They usually form a useful adjunct to other qualitative methods, such as interviews, where they help to corroborate claims made in interview or locate exact dates of key events. They may also be used as the central data source, particularly for historical events. Documents can be analysed both qualitatively and quantitatively. Another hypothetical example may help to illustrate the process of devising and selecting an appropriate methodology.

If the research question focused on the role of the SCP in attaining prescribing rights for podiatrists, how would the study be designed? As you are not attempting to intervene to make change, but to explore and understand what has been happening, a qualitative design may again be appropriate. Clearly interviews with present and past members of Council and the Medicines Committee would be relevant, as would interviews with present and past officials within the Medicines and Healthcare Products Regulatory Agency (and its predecessors, the Medicines Control Agency and Medicines Commission). Perhaps those within the Department of Health or other professional or regulatory bodies would be appropriate subjects.

Finding new evidence – research design

Interviews in these circumstances would necessarily involve accounts of various meetings within and between organisations, but it would be unreasonable to expect respondents to remember the exact dates and sequences of these meetings, especially over a long timeframe. Therefore, documents could provide this data and add to the clarity and understanding of what occurred. Minutes of meetings help to corroborate (triangulate) interview accounts, as do memoranda, emails and personal letters. Sequencing events can also be constructed by looking at consultation letters (known as MLXs), health service circulars, government White Papers and Statutory Instruments and their associated Acts of Parliament. These enable the researcher to trace the sequence of official events, grasp the content of proceedings and triangulate other sources of data. They give a context to the events but they do need to be interpreted with care – and key actors can be very helpful in assisting with this process.

As prescribing in podiatry is not new, but part of an ongoing process over several decades, documents can help to provide a record of the timings and sequence of events over long time periods. Particular perspectives will also be captured in this way. For example, analysing the content of the SCP journals may highlight official views from the SCP regarding progress or obstacles to progress. They may indicate professional responses to official Department of Health policy and allow a picture of strategic intent to be constructed over time.

For most contemporaneous periods, documentary sources tend to be supplemented by, or are an adjunct to, interviews or other sources of data, and are crucial to adequate triangulation.

Observation

Participant observation

Observation is another qualitative means of gathering data which is popular within disciplines such as anthropology and sociology and it has gained popularity with nursing researchers in recent years. It may involve either participant observational techniques, which means that the researcher becomes an active participant in the events he or she is studying, or it may be confined to non-participant observation, where the researcher observes events from the sidelines. In terms of research design, this would be an appropriate method to use where the research question seeks to uncover what people did in a particular environment or circumstance, rather than what they said they would do. One of the disadvantages of relying on people's stated opinions about a particular situation is that they often say one thing and do another when faced with the situation in reality.

Participant observation involves immersing yourself in the group you are studying, as if becoming part of it. It may involve letting the group know that you are there as an observer (the usual participant observer status) or trying to become part of the group covertly (being a complete participant observer). This may or may not be difficult, depending on the group in question, and that will determine whether or not it is feasible to attempt that method. For example, you may pass as a legitimate member of a local SCP branch, if that group were your chosen research focus, but blending into a group of consultant podiatric surgeons (if you are not one yourself) may prove a little harder, due to their specialist knowledge and experiences. There are also, of course, ethical problems associated with covert research.

Quantitative research designs

Quantitative designs

A quantitative research study typically has a very specific research question, such as does medicament A reduce/cure fungal nail infections? In quantitative research methods, the researcher often defines a null hypothesis of no change, in this case that medicament A will not have an effect on fungal nail growth, and then, through the research study, aims to disprove this null hypothesis. This is a conservative approach which ensures that decisions are taken that change the status quo only if there is sufficient evidence to show that the status quo is wrong. During the research project one variable or a number of variables will be manipulated to test the hypothesis. In this example, the independent variable is medicament A and the dependent variable is fungal nail growth, as by manipulating the independent variable (medicament) an effect may be shown on the dependent variable (fungal growth).

There are many types of quantitative research designs, with varying degrees of scientific rigour. Systematic reviews [5] or

Finding new evidence – research design

Randomised controlled trials (RCTs) [6] are believed to provide the highest quality of evidence (Level 1 studies). The Centre for Reviews and Dissemination [7] uses the following five levels of research design, in descending order of strength of evidence:

1. Experimental studies (RCTs)
2. Quasi-experimental studies (no randomisation)
3. Controlled observation studies with control groups (cohort or case control)
4. Observation studies without control groups
5. Expert opinion based on pathophysiology, bench research or consensus.

Systematic reviews

Systematic reviews

Systematic reviews group together all the studies available on a particular topic, such as treatment for fungal nail infections, and critically appraise and summarise all the research on this topic which meets the appropriate standard. This type of review of the literature uses highly standardised review methodology. Statistical methods (meta-analysis) may also be used to analyse and summarise the results of the included studies. Therefore, the evidence from a systematic review may be stronger as it is based on a number of studies, and a greater number of interventions and subjects will be included.

Randomised controlled trials (RCTs)

RCTs

RCTs are often used when testing a new treatment, and involve randomly allocating the sample group to the treatment arm of the study (where they receive the new treatment under test) or a control area. Randomisation of patients to either group can be done in a number of ways (for example, using postcodes or random number tables) and ensures that there are no systematic differences in the patient groups receiving each kind of treatment. The participants in the control arm should ideally receive only a placebo treatment or no intervention, to compare against the active treatment.

However, there are practical and ethical problems in

withholding treatment for research purposes and it is more usual to compare the effects of a new treatment to the best treatment currently available. In our example of the fungal nail infections, a control group would indicate whether mycotic nail infections resolve without any intervention and could separate out the effect of the natural history of the condition from the additional effect of the medicament.

Ideally, neither the researcher nor study participants should be aware of which treatment each study participant is receiving (this is called a double blind trial). If this is not possible, then the participants must be unaware (single blind). This is important as the effects observed should be solely the result of the intervention being assessed, and not because the study participants know what they have been given and react accordingly. True blinding is often difficult to achieve in practice.

An example

As an example of a quantitative research design, let us use the previous example of assessing whether medicament A is a useful treatment for fungal nail infections. (We will assume that there is no current evidence for effective topical treatment so that using a control group receiving no treatment is ethical.)

Three groups of patients could be recruited to the study: Group 1 who apply medicament A to their nails as directed; Group 2 who apply an identical-looking, but inert, placebo medicament; and Group 3 who do not have any intervention (control group). Other confounding variables may need to be taken into account that could affect the results, such as age, sex and ethnicity of the study participants, whether they have had previous treatment for their nail condition, whether they are taking other medications, whether they suffer from medical problems that may affect the use of the drug, how long the fungal nail infection has been present, what type of infection it is and the amount of nail that has been affected. To ensure that such variables do not affect the results, you should ensure that each group has similar representation from particular age groups, genders, ethnic groups and so on.

The number of patients required for each group should be determined before the study begins. It is usually based on the size of the difference being measured, the variability of the outcome measures and the statistical tests used (and needs to be decided with the help of a statistician). How fungal nail infection is to be measured (the outcome) should also be considered. This could be done with a matrix placed over the nail to assess the area of nail affected. However, if a number of researchers are involved, a guide to ensure that researchers all measure in the same way (inter-rater reliability) should be considered. How long will the study last? Will the participants be assessed for fungal nail involvement only at the end of the study, regularly throughout the study, or at the beginning and end of the study?

This study may use a pre- and post-test, where the degree of nail affected by a fungus is assessed at the beginning and end of the study in each of the three groups. Most quantitative research studies use statistical tests to show whether a difference has occurred and, if it has, how likely it is that this effect could have happened purely by chance. You should consult a statistician before undertaking a research project to discuss the type of statistical test required and the numbers of study participants necessary to measure a change. They can also advise on appropriate research design.

Guiding principles of research design

Guiding principles

Design is critical to the success of research and will determine whether it is possible to provide answers to the research questions posed. Robson [8] suggests that a qualitative research design requires: a conceptual framework, research question(s), a sampling strategy and decisions on methods and data collection tools. Each of these issues has been addressed above, with some examples used to illustrate the key points. He also asserts that the research design provides the link between the research question(s), the data collected and the conclusions that are drawn. The research design is, essentially, the research plan. It is about planning the right type and combination of methods to obtain the right data to answer the research questions posed at the start of the study.

Each variation of qualitative and quantitative designs will have its particular requirements. When conducting any research project, choosing the most appropriate design to answer the research question is the most important factor. Other practical considerations include the amount of time available, the cost of the study, whether the appropriate number of patients can be recruited and the number of researchers needed to carry out the investigation.

Sometimes consideration of these factors will mean that you have to modify the original design, or ask a more focused question. It is important, however, that you understand and anticipate the effects of any modification of the design, otherwise the findings of the study may be invalidated or may not provide sufficient evidence to answer your research question. It is vital that you seek expert advice on the design of any research project at an early stage.

References

[1] D. L. Lorimer. A Short History of the Society of Chiropodists and Podiatrists 1945–1995. *Journal of British Podiatric Medicine*, 50.5 (1995) Supplement, 25.

[2] C. Hine. *Issues in Social Research on the Internet* (Oxford: Berg, 2005).

[3] C. Mann and F. Stewart. *Internet Communication and Qualitative Research: A handbook for researching online* (London: Sage, 2000).

[4] J. Scott *A Matter of Record: Documentary sources in social research* (Cambridge: Polity Press, 1990).

[5] National Health and Medical Research Council. *Guidelines for the Development and Implementation of Clinical Guidelines* (Canberra: Australian Government Publishing Service, 1995).

[6] G. Guyatt, D. Sackett, J. Sinclair, R. Hayward, D. Cook and R. Cook. Users' Guides to the Medical Literature – IX: A method for grading healthcare recommendations. *The Journal of the American Medical Association*, **274** (1995), 1800–4.

[7] NHS Centre for Reviews and Dissemination. *Undertaking Systematic Reviews of Research on Effectiveness: CRD guidelines for those carrying out or commissioning reviews* (York: University of York, 1996).

[8] C. Robson. *Real World Research – A resource for social scientists* (Oxford: Blackwell, 1993).

Chapter 5
Action research
Wesley Vernon

Action research is a relatively informal, but potentially extremely useful, research technique, which has been used infrequently in podiatry to date. It is a process which neatly links day-to-day actions with research and allows changes to be made and understanding to be gained at the same time. As such, it should have great relevance at the point of delivery of a service and should be of genuine practical value. Action research has been defined in various ways:

- a form of self-reflective enquiry by participants, undertaken in order to improve understanding of their practices in context with a view to maximising social justice [1]

- a process by which change and understanding can be pursued at the one time [2]

- a research paradigm which allows you to develop knowledge or understanding as part of practice. [3]

All these have the components of a task, action or change process, and reflection or understanding. Simply put, the process is a quest for knowledge about how to improve.

Importantly, action research is a cyclical process for which a model of understanding has been developed. This model has four main components, as shown in Figure 5.1 (below).

Figure 5.1
The action research cycle

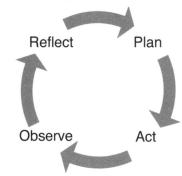

Reflect Plan

Observe Act

It is, however, more of a spiral than a cyclical process, because as one cycle of action research has been completed, improved understanding then leads to further planning and action and so on. Figure 5.1 shows the full action research model, but it can be simplified further, as shown in Figure 5.2 (below).

Figure 5.2

A simplified action research cycle

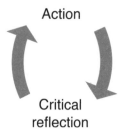

Action

Critical reflection

It is a natural process of alternating action and reflection. The reflection period will cover considerations such as: how well did the action go? what was good or not so good? what has been learned? how could it have been done better? and so on. This will then lead to improved understanding, with conclusions being derived from the exercise and, from these, plans for further actions can be prepared and undertaken.

Many people may feel that they already work in this way. The difference lies in the rigour with which the planning, and especially the reflection, are approached. With action research, frequent in-depth critical assessment should take place, with special attention to aspects of the action which may have produced unexpected results. There is more systematic collection of evidence and problems are posed and considered in addition to dealing with those that are there to be solved. It also requires collaboration. It is not research that is simply 'done to other people', but a process which requires active participation from the researcher and everyone involved.

Historical overview

Historical overview

Action research was founded by Kurt Lewin (1948), an American social psychologist and educator [4]. He used the term to describe work which did not separate research investigations from the action needed to solve a problem. Lewin believed that research should not be undertaken as a theoretical academic exercise but applied in the real world (echoing Karl Marx who famously wrote, a century earlier, that the task of philosophy should not simply be to understand the world, but to change it).

One of the first people to use action research was Stephen Correy at a teaching college in the US [5]. He saw that action research had a more direct effect on particular practice than other forms of generalised research. Correy also noted that collaboration was essential in the action research process. In the 1950s, however, action research was widely attacked as being unscientific and quantitative research methodologies predominated.

Much later, in the 1970s, educationalists noted that quantitative experiments were of little relevance to their own day-to-day work and could not resolve their particular issues and problems. Action research again emerged in teaching and was found to be extremely useful. Through this interest, action research was widely adopted by the teaching profession and many different applications were identified.

Strengths

Strengths

Action research has a number of advantages. Firstly, it is simple to perform. It is not a complex esoteric research method requiring statistical knowledge or complex qualitative language. It is a development of a natural process and anyone can do it. A prior research design is not needed and the process can be worked out as the research proceeds. The method is less likely to fail as a research approach because it offers a high degree of flexibility in implementation.

It is also cost-effective and practical to perform. It will not require large-scale research funding to be implemented and can simply be performed as a series of workplace-based meetings with follow-up tasks. In addition, as a natural everyday process, the approach may not require ethical approval (but this will be worth checking with local research advisers depending on the proposal to be considered). In the past, I have taken some action research projects to ethical committees to be told that ethical approval was unnecessary while other projects have been considered to require ethical approval. For still other studies, the general opinion has been that a 'project' was being undertaken, rather than research. The reality is that much of the teaching profession is routinely using action research for continuing professional development (CPD). Under the new ethical arrangements, it would not be practically possible for ethics committees to consider all of these cases. However, if you are in any doubt, you should seek approval.

Secondly, action research is a tool for change. As such, it overcomes the perceived persistent failure of research to impact on and improve practice. This is one of the main purposes of action research and part of its philosophical underpinnings. As such, action research focuses on issues pertinent to the researcher and is also therefore directly relevant to the workplace. In turn, it should bring direct improvement for the organisation involved.

Thirdly, action research has strong communication benefits. It not only bridges the gap between management and workers through direct involvement, but can also bridge similar or even wider gaps between organisations and patients. Communication benefits can also include communications within wider networks, in addition to those in the immediate workplace.

Finally, action research is a learning process. The critical reflection involved offers many opportunities to remedy problems or errors, and any prior assumptions in the area in question are tested in action. The improved knowledge gained allows much opportunity for self-reflection, which in turn brings improvements in self-awareness. In all the action research projects I have experienced, every participant (including myself) has learned much from the process.

Criticisms and limitations

Criticisms and limitations

All is not perfect, however, and there are a number of limitations to action research, which need to be understood if you are planning to use the techniques.

Unlike other research methods, action research is often of value only to the researcher and his or her work environment, with the findings not being generalisable beyond the immediate setting. This is not always the case. Sometimes findings can be generalisable either in terms of theory, or, less frequently, data, but it is important to realise that this will not necessarily be so.

Action research can require much time and energy – more so than simply doing the everyday task being investigated. Therefore, it is important to keep your feet on the ground and not become over-ambitious in the changes you attempt to make through the process. This effect can also be compounded by a general resistance to change, which, if present, can hamper the researcher's efforts, in terms of gaining access to files, other data and clinics for observation.

Importantly, action research is not seen as 'real research' by some authorities (even by qualitative research authorities who have had to fend off criticisms of their own research approaches from the quantitative research camp over the years). While the criticisms of the 1950s have been mainly refuted, it has been said that there remains a problem of 'data, which can make no claim to be generally representative' [6]. In other words, the field of action research shows how to collect the data, but not how that data could, or should, be handled.

In the strictest sense, the wider community should be able to validate a study, not just the researcher who carried it out. If such work is believed to be of relevance chiefly to the researcher and his or her team, then findings which are meaningful, and therefore useful to the researcher, could be discussed with colleagues, mentors, patients or focus groups, or written up as a case study for a professional journal.

Why action research is useful to podiatrists

Why action research is useful

Action research should be useful to podiatry in many respects. The following areas are some in which this approach could be useful but this list is by no means exhaustive.

Podiatry education and development

Podiatry is experiencing many developmental changes at present and practitioners are having to learn new concepts and translate these into clinical practice for the first time. An action research approach can help with this process. Similarly, action research has been used in teaching for CPD purposes for many years and there would be a benefit for the reflective podiatrist in undertaking personal action research to enhance their own personal development.

Management

Action research could have wide value in podiatry management. The NHS is in a process of change and change management facilitation is one of the main values of action research. Not only could it be used to initiate change but also to gain ownership and agreement of required changes in order to smooth the process of change as it takes place. Amongst other management uses, action research could be used by podiatrists for personal evaluation as part of annual appraisal and self-monitoring purposes.

Research

Finally, action research is a research technique and as such could be useful to podiatry departments who wish to undertake research for a variety of reasons.

How to go about action research

How to go about it

So how do you go about undertaking action research when you may have had little involvement in research of any type? Here are a few suggestions.

Implementation

- Put a small group together and learn through doing action research.
- Start with a short-term simple project before taking on more complex issues.
- Organise the group to work to a realistic, but efficient, time schedule.
- Build reflection and discussion time into the planned group activity.
- Where necessary include those involved in the action (certainly staff, but also perhaps patients)

Consensus research techniques can be useful in an action research approach. However, they can be much more complex to perform than basic action research, so, for the first-time researcher, these are best avoided.

Group activity

- Take care with the group dynamics. It is important not to be intolerant with the group members as the group will only work well in a relaxed atmosphere.
- Monitor activity throughout the research process and keep detailed notes throughout.
- Keep a constant check that the project is improving your practice in line with your personal values.
- Maintain a flexible approach.

Questions to use

Questions used in action research should be:

- complex (not simply inviting yes/no answers)
- couched in simple language
- concise
- meaningful
- without a known, correct answer
- about something over which the researcher has an influence.

Data sources

There is a wide range of data sources that could be used as part of an action research project. These might include:

- new data (e.g. interviews, focus groups, questionnaires, surveys)
- existing data (e.g. records, files, memos, meeting notes, case studies)
- reflections (e.g. diaries, self-assessments, field notes).

These sources might be in a variety of different formats (e.g. audio tape, video, pictures and text).

Data should be appropriate, easy to collect, and accessible, and at least two sources should be used for each piece of information, so that triangulation checks can be made.

Interpretation

- Organise data into trends and themes.
- Use collected data and current literature to plan the course of action of the research.

Evaluation

When evaluating the results of the change implemented, consider:

- Has an improvement occurred?
- Does evidence demonstrate the improvement?
- If not, what changes could show better results?

Act on the findings

This is the spiral of action research which can continue as long as the researcher is interested or able.

An example

The following is an example of the action research process.

- *Research question:* In a really busy clinic setting, what can I do to ensure that high-priority patients can still get appointments at short notice?
- *Reflect:* Is this a problem at the moment and how do I know? (Keep and examine clinic data to monitor.) How is the diary kept at present? Is there anything in the literature to suggest better or different systems?
- *Plan:* Get a small group together. Brainstorm to prepare and consider the options for change. Agree the most viable option. Discuss and agree the process of implementation.
- *Act:* Implement and communicate the change, following the agreed plan.
- *Observe:* What happens? What changes have occurred? Does it work? What are the problems? What do the patients think about the change?
- *Reflect:* What benefits have resulted? How could this have been done better? What was learned from the experience? Was this worth doing, or were things better before? How do we know that this was an improvement? How do the findings compare with the literature? What else needs doing that is related? How could this best be followed up?
- *Write up your conclusions.*

References

[1] W. Carr and S. Kemmis. *Becoming Critical: Education, knowledge and action research* (Lewes: Falmer, 1986).

[2] B. Dick. *Action Learning and Action Research*. Available at www.scu.edu.au/schools/gcm/ar/arhome.html. Accessed on 15.12.06.

[3] B. Dick and P. Swepson. *Action Research FAQ*. Available at www.scu.edu.au/schools/gcm/ar/arhome.html. Accessed on 15.12.06.

[4] K. Lewin. Resolving social conflicts. In *Selected Papers on Group Dynamics*, ed. G. W. Lewin (New York: Harper & Row, 1948).

[5] S. M. Correy. Action research, fundamental research and educational practices. *Teachers College Record,* 50 (1949), 509–14.

[6] L. Cohen, L. Manion and K. Morrison. *Research Methods in Education*, 5th edn (London: Routledge/Falmer, 2000).

Further reading

There are many resources available for those interested in undertaking action research. Two that are particularly useful are:

L. Cohen, L. Manion and K. Morrison. *Research Methods in Education*, 5th edn (London: Routledge/Falmer, 2000). This contains an excellent overview of action research and is useful to give the reader a basic working knowledge of the approaches.

B. Dick. Action Research Resources website. Available at www.scu.edu.au/schools/gcm/ar/arhome.html.
This website is maintained by Bob Dick. It contains information and links to relevant journals, courses, other action research websites, mailing lists, action research institutes, papers, dissertations, work in progress and conference abstracts. Thes are substantial and useful resources both to those new to action research and those with wide experience.

Chapter 6
Data collection
Lisa Farndon and Alan Borthwick

Previous chapters have discussed research design and, in particular, action research. This chapter builds on these by looking at some of the ways in which the data needed for a variety of research designs can be collected and considers some of the important features of data collection methods.

Data characteristics

The collection of data is the vital link in the research process between asking the research question (and designing the research study) and finding the answers. If the data collected is unreliable, inaccurate or does not represent what you wanted to measure then, at best, the results will be meaningless and, at worst, could be misleading or wrong. The key to collecting good data is in defining appropriate measures. Good research design should ensure that the data is collected in a way that does not bias the results and does answer the questions.

Data can take many different forms and the sort of data that is collected is determined by the type of study and the information required. For example, in a study investigating why new patients seek podiatry care [1], a qualitative line of enquiry was adopted, the data collected was from verbal experiences and opinions and the data collection method used was a semi-structured interview. However, a randomised trial investigating the efficacy of exercise therapy and orthoses in the treatment of knee pain [2] used quantitative measures: a pain visual analogue scale (VAS) in conjunction with two knee pain scales.

The basic requirements of good data are reliability and validity. Reliability refers to the consistency of the data and, in quantitative methodologies, usually means how repeatable the data are. Validity refers to the accuracy of the data (does it actually measure what it has been designed to measure?). Data can be reliable but not valid (for example, repeated weighings on bathroom scales with little variation where the zero point was not set correctly) or valid but not reliable (for example, scales with a correctly set zero point where the recorded weight is highly dependent on where you stand, so there is a great deal of variation in repeated weighings).

In qualitative methodologies, these two characteristics take on rather different, but related meanings. The concepts of reliability and validity are harder to define in qualitative research and may be best expressed as credibility (how truthful is the data?), transferability (would similar data be meaningful in different contexts?), dependability (could the findings be replicated in identical situations?) and confirmability (can researcher bias be ruled out?) [3].

Measurement tools

Measurement tools

Measurement tools (or instruments) are the mechanisms which enable data to be collected. They can range from simple mechanical instruments such as a goniometer to measure joint angles or a 10 g monofilament to assess cutaneous sense to more complex devices such as force platforms and in-shoe pressure sensors. However, the term is also used to include ways of capturing other information such as questionnaire-based indices (for example, quality of life measurement using the SF-36 or pain assessment using the McGill pain questionnaire).

Any measurement tool should be consistent (reliable), such that the same score would result if the measurement were repeated on the same patient at the same time. A test-retest reliability exercise can be used to assess the stability of an instrument. Here the researcher will use the instrument on a number of patients at different times to see whether the results are consistent.

Measurement tools also have to be accurate (valid) and should be tested to show this. Three separate criteria are often examined during the validation process. These are content validity (do the items in an instrument reflect the subject under investigation?), construct validity (does the instrument measure the subject under investigation?) and internal consistency (do items correlate well with each other and with the total questionnaire score?) [4].

Outcome measures in podiatry

Outcome measures

Assessment of the effect of a particular treatment is an important factor in podiatry care and a number of specific podiatric outcome measures have therefore been developed.

The **Foot Function Index** (FFI) was formulated and validated by Budiman-Mak *et al.* [5] to assess the functional impact of foot pathologies in terms of pain, disability and activity restriction. It consists of a self-administered questionnaire with 23 items divided into three sub-sections and was first used on patients with rheumatoid arthritis. The scoring system is based on the supposition that the number of situations in which an individual experiences pain, difficulty or limited activity due to a foot problem, in combination with the intensity of that experience in each situation, determines how severely foot function is impaired. Therefore, the higher the FFI score, the greater the impairment. This index was later evaluated in a study comparing the FFI scores of both feet (side-to-side reliability) in 30 people with rheumatoid arthritis and was found to be a reliable tool [6].

The **Foot Health Status Questionnaire** (FHSQ) is designed to measure foot health-related quality of life and consists of three sections: a measure of foot health from a score of 0 (representing poor foot health) to a score of 100 (for optimum foot health), a generic measure of health based on the Short Form 36 (SF-36) quality of life questionnaire [7] and some demographic measures, such as socio-economic status and satisfaction [8].

The FHSQ was compared with the FFI by Bennet and Patterson [8] on 111 subjects who completed both questionnaires. A subsequent clinical examination found the FHSQ was a more suitable measure than the FFI, as it could help researchers identify changes in foot health status resulting from a therapeutic or surgical intervention. Landorf and Keenan [9] also compared the two measures to assess the effectiveness of foot orthoses in people with plantar fasciitis. They also found that the FHSQ was more sensitive in measuring health-related quality of life in this client group and recommended this should be the preferred choice when assessing the effectiveness of foot orthoses. The outcomes of podiatric surgery in 140 patients were investigated using the FHSQ [10] and it was suggested that surgery gave favourable results for patients in relation to pain, physical function and improved general foot health. Positive results were also found in a similar study conducted in the UK measuring FHSQ scores before and after podiatric surgery, demonstrating comparable results in all but one criterion [11].

More patient-centred measures

More patient-centred measures

Some measures have been developed which are more patient centred. Garrow [4] has developed and validated a tool to measure foot pain and disability that is sensitive to individuals with a range of different problems affecting mobility (the **Manchester Foot Pain and Disability Questionnaire**). It comprises 19 questions relating to daily activities and asks about pain experienced whilst conducting these, during the past month. There are three responses: 'none of the time', 'on some days' or 'on most/every day'. This measure has been recommended for use in a variety of clinical and population settings and was later used by Waxman and colleagues [12] in a randomised controlled trial (RCT) measuring the effect of a self-care foot programme for older people.

The **Podiatry Health Questionnaire** (PHQ) consists of both a questionnaire which the patient completes regarding the effect their foot health has on their quality of life and a clinical measure (on a scale from one to five, five reflecting gross foot problems) which is completed by the podiatrist [13]. This measure was piloted in individuals across four UK podiatry departments and was found to be a useful tool to assess foot-related health.

The **Foot Impact Scale** [14] is based on the results of patient interviews and a postal survey. It consists of a 51-item questionnaire investigating impairments, footwear, activities and participation. Initial results suggest that the tool has external validity and is reliable.

The **Bristol Foot Score** [15] was also formulated after patient consultations, with groups of patients and on an individual basis, and consists of 15 items with various responses for each. Each answer is scored, the total score is calculated and the higher the final score, the more significant an individual perceives their foot problem to be. It involves three inter-related topics: foot pain, footwear and general foot health. Once developed, it was used to assess outcomes of nail surgery and found that the pre- and post-operative scores for the sample group showed a significant difference (the post-operative scores being lower), suggesting nail surgery was beneficial.

Questionnaires and surveys

Surveys

Surveys can be used to elicit information from a sample of the population. They are a popular research tool in podiatry and have been used widely to determine the incidence of foot problems in different populations [16,17], to assess a variety of professional issues [18,19] and to gauge the effectiveness of specific podiatric interventions [20, 21]. Surveys are often in the form of a self-administered questionnaire [22], but can also be conducted by interview where the researcher asks a number of pre-determined questions and records the responses. A number of advantages and disadvantages are associated with the use of different survey methods.

Face-to-face interviews, following a fixed format, can allow more complex data to be collected as the interviewer is on hand to clarify any problems. Open-ended questions can be asked [23] and response rates are often higher when compared with postal surveys. Telephone interviews are cheap and quick to administer when compared with face-to-face interviews. However, those without a telephone will automatically be excluded from the survey, which could introduce an element of bias.

Postal surveys, using a self-completed questionnaire, are probably the most common as they are cheap to administer when compared with face-to-face interviews and can cover a large geographical area. They eliminate the potential for interviewer bias and they avoid the problem of the respondents being unavailable for interview [23]. However, Bourque and Fielder [24] recommend using an accurate and current list of the population under study before a sampling frame is determined. Response rates are also generally lower than in face-to-face and telephone interviews, allowing non-response bias to be a potential problem although reminders can lessen this [25]. It is recommended that postal survey questionnaires should be short and easy to complete without the assistance of others [24], although there is no guarantee that other members of the household will not complete the questionnaire on behalf of the respondent.

The actual format of questionnaires has been discussed widely in the literature, especially the issue of the inclusion of 'don't know' or a neutral response. Some authors recommend the omission of this response category as it does not affect response rates, presents a questionnaire in a simpler format [26] and avoids the respondent opting for the middle ground [27]. Hawkins and Coney [28] however, advocate the use of a 'don't know' option to reduce the rate of uninformed responses.

Response order has also been shown to affect survey results. Primacy effects, where the first category is preferentially selected, and recency effects, where the last option is picked more often, have been shown to occur in all types of surveys, although Schuman and Presser [29] believe that primacy effects may be more likely to occur in postal surveys. To avoid this, it has been suggested to change the order of response categories for each question, although this can make completion of the questionnaire more time-consuming. When given a statement which requires agreement or disagreement, Ayidiya and McClendon [30] found that agreement would be higher if the statement was written in a forced choice format; this is known as the 'acquiescence effect'. A space for free comments alongside each question has also been found to increase response rates [31].

Qualitative data collection methods

Data collection

The most common ways of collecting qualitative data are by one-to-one interviews, focus groups or by collecting textual information in the form of documents. (The available methods are listed in more detail in Chapter 4.)

When using interviews as a data collection method, the interaction between the researcher and participant is usually taped and later transcribed verbatim. This can be supplemented with notes that the researcher may make during, or directly after, the interview (field notes), which capture any ideas or thoughts that may have occurred which could aid the analysis and interpretation of data. During the analysis stage, narrative data is coded into themes, which can be compared across the different participants who took part in the study.

Focus groups can be taped and later transcribed, but as they can consist of up to ten people with numerous interactions, this can be quite difficult to record accurately and later transcribe. To improve this method, an additional researcher can be included, alongside the facilitator of the group, to make notes during the exchanges, noting any particular themes, issues or relevant details. If researchers have a lot of experience in running focus groups, they may just collect data by note taking. Using more than one researcher to do this, who can then compare their notes at a later date, can improve the reliability of this method.

When using documentary data, one of the most important considerations is to ensure that all the relevant documents are assembled. An incomplete record might bias the findings. If large numbers of documents are involved, which could not possibly be analysed in a realistic timeframe, then a random sample of the available material is advised. Rodgers [32] advises retrieving a 20 per cent sample when using concept analysis, a qualitative research method used widely in nursing. Once an appropriate sample of material has been collated, this information is then ordered into themes and analysed.

Conclusion

There are a wide variety of data collection methods available to the podiatry profession. These can range from simple ways of assessing the efficacy of a treatment, such as assessing the reduction in the size of lesions or their resolution [33], investigating the success and any potential complications of podiatric surgery using the PASCOM system [34] or by utilising a previously validated measure to assess changes in foot health as a result of a podiatric intervention. Discussion with patients, carers and professionals, in the form of focus groups and interviews, can also yield important information regarding service delivery [18] and professional issues [35].

The vital characteristics of effective data collection are that the data should be reliable and valid and these terms may be interpreted in different ways to reflect the research design being used. The aims and objectives of a project or research study should determine which type of data collection method is used.

References

[1] L. J. Farndon, D. W. Vernon, S. Morris, K. Littlewood, A. Barnes and J. Burnside. Why do New Patients Seek NHS Podiatry Care? A multi-centre qualitative study. *British Journal of Podiatry*, **7**.1 (2004), 17–20.

[2] S. Wiener-Ogilvie and R. B. Jones. A randomised trial of exercise therapy and foot orthoses as treatment for knee pain in primary care. *British Journal of Podiatry*, **7**.2 (2004), 43–9.

[3] N. Fox. Data collection by observation. In *Research Approaches in Primary Care*, eds. A. Wilson, M. Williams and B. Hancock (Oxford: Radcliffe Medical Press, 2000).

[4] A. P. Garrow, A. C. Papageorgiou, A. J.Silman, E. Thomas, M. I. Jayson and G. J. Macfarlane. Development and validation of a questionnaire to assess disabling foot pain. *Pain*, **85** (2000), 107–13.

[5] E. Budiman-Mak, K. J. Conrad and K. E. Roach. The Foot Function Index: A measure of foot pain and disability. *Journal of Clinical Epidemiology*, **44** (1991), 561–70.

[6] K. G. Saag, C. L. Saltzman, C. K. Brown and E. Budiman-Mak. The Foot Function Index for Measuring Rheumatoid Arthritis Pain: Evaluating side-to-side reliability. *Foot & Ankle International,* **17** (1996), 506–10.

[7] J. Ware and C. Sherbourne. The MOS 36-item Short-Form Health Survey 1: Conceptual framework and item selection. *Medical Care*, **30** (1992), 473–83.

[8] P. J. Bennett and C. Patterson. The Foot Health Status Questionnaire (FHSQ): A new instrument for measuring outcomes of footcare. *Australasian Journal of Podiatric Medicine*, **32** (1998), 87–92.

[9] K. Landorf and A. Keenan. An evaluation of two foot-specific, health-related quality-of-life measuring instruments. *Foot and Ankle International*, **23** (2002), 538–46.

[10] P. J. Bennett, C. Patterson and M. P. Dunne. Health-related quality of life following podiatric surgery. *Journal of the American Podiatric Medical Association,* **91** (2001), 164–73.

[11] P. J. Claisse, L. A. Jones and R. Mehta. Reporting Foot Surgery Outcomes in Every-day Practice: Using a foot-related quality of life measure. *British Journal of Podiatry*, **8** (2005), 112–17.

[12] R. Waxman, H. Woodburn, M. Powell, J. Woodburn, S. Blackburn and P. Helliwell. FOOTSTEP: A randomized controlled trial investigating the clinical and cost effectiveness of a patient self-management programme for basic foot care in the elderly. *Journal of Clinical Epidemiology*, 56 (2003), 1092–9.

[13] S. Macran, P. Kind, J. Collingwood, R. Hull, I. McDonald and L. Parkinson. Evaluating Podiatry Services: Testing a treatment specific measure of health status. *Quality of Life Research*, 12 (2003), 177–88.

[14] P. Helliwell, N. Reay, G. Gilworth, A. Redmond, A. Slade and A. Tennant A. Development of a foot impact scale for rheumatoid arthritis. *Arthritis & Rheumatism*, 53 (2005), 418–22.

[15] S. Barnett, R. Campbell and I. Harvey. The Bristol Foot Score: Developing a patient-based foot-health measure. *Journal of the American Podiatric Medical Association*, 95 (2005), 264–72.

[16] L. A. Levy. Prevalence of Chronic Podiatric Conditions in the US: National Health Survey 1990. *Journal of the American Podiatric Medical Association*, 82 (1992), 221–3.

[17] L. Merriman. What is the Purpose of Chiropody Services? *Journal of British Podiatric Medicine*, 48 (1993), 121–8.

[18] E. MacDonald and S. Capewell. Podiatry: Cinderella speciality in search of a glass slipper. *Podiatry Now*, 4 (2001), 518–20.

[19] L. Farndon and S. Nancarrow. Employment and career development opportunities for podiatrists and foot care assistants in the NHS. *British Journal of Podiatry*, 6 (2003), 103–8.

[20] M. Price, J. Tasker, N. Taylor and T. Sheeran. Not Just a Piece of Plastic? A survey of orthoses effectiveness within a podiatric surgery department. *British Journal of Podiatry*, 5 (2002), 36–40.

[21] J. Walter Jr., G. Ng and J. Stoltz. A patient satisfaction survey on prescription custom-molded foot orthoses. *Journal of the American Podiatric Medical Association*, 94 (2004), 363–7.

[22] D. F. Polit and B. P. Hungler. *Nursing Research: Principles and methods* (Philadelphia: Lippincott, 1999).

[23] E. McColl, A. Jacoby, L. Thomas, J. Soutter, C. Bamford and N. Steen. Design and Use of Questionnaires: A review of best practice applicable to surveys of health service staff and patients. *Health Technology Assessment*, 5.31 (2001).

[24] L. Bourque and E. Fielder. *How to Conduct Self-administered Mail Surveys* (Thousand Oaks, CA: Sage, 1995).

[25] C. Moser and G. Kalton. *Survey Methods in Social Investigation* (Aldershot: Gower, 1971).

[26] G. Poe, I. Seeman, J. McLaughlin, E. Mehl and M. Dietz. 'Don't know' Boxes in Factual Questions in a Mail Questionnaire: Effects on level and quality of response. *Public Opinion Quarterly*, 52 (1988), 212–22.

[27] G. Bishop. Experiments with the Middle Response Alternative in Survey Questions. *Public Opinion Quarterly*, 51 (1987), 220–32.

[28] D. Hawkins and K. Coney. Uninformed Response Error in Survey Research. *Journal of Marketing Research*, 18 (1981), 370–4.

[29] H. Schuman and S. Presser. *Questions and Answers in Attitude Surveys: Experiments on question form, wording and content* (New York: Academic Press, 1981).

[30] S. Ayidiya and M. McClendon. Response Effects in Mail Surveys. *Public Opinion Quarterly*, 54 (1990), 229–47.

[31] A. Trice and M. Dolan. Hotel ratings vs effects of format and survey length. *Psychological Reports*, 56 (1985), 176–8.

[33] B. Rodgers. Concept Analysis: An evolutionary view. In *Concept Development in Nursing: Foundations, techniques and applications*, eds. B. Rodgers and K. Knafl (Philadelphia: Saunders, 2000).

[34] L. Farndon and L. Marriot. An Alternative Method for Treating Painful Corns: A two centre audit. *Podiatry Now*, 5 (2002), 225–8.

[35] G. Rudge and D. Tollafield. A critical assessment of a new evaluation tool for podiatric surgical outcome analysis. *British Journal of Podiatry*, 6 (2003), 109–19.

[36] A. Borthwick and T. Clarke. Registration and 'Grandparenting' in Podiatry: Non-registrant practitioners' views. *British Journal of Podiatry*, 7 (2004), 71–6.

Chapter 7
Finding the funding for research
Farina Hashmi

One additional vital component of the research process is gaining sufficient financial support for the research proposed. This article indicates the main sources of research funding and support that are available to Allied Health Professionals (AHPs) and some valuable pointers when preparing an application for funding. Specific funding opportunities do appear and disappear, however, and some of the grants mentioned below may change over time. You should always seek current information and advice and there is a list of useful websites that you can refer to at the end of the chapter.

Sources of funding

Sources of funding

There are a variety of funding organisations in the UK specifically geared towards clinical research. In the past, high profile research councils (such as the Medical Research Council) and charities (such as Diabetes UK) have focused mainly on supporting basic science research and clinical trials in medicine. Although organisations such as the Medical Research Council and the Wellcome Trust do support health research, competition for these grants is strong, particularly with current trends in basic science leaning heavily towards stem cell research.

The Department of Health (DH) awards a high proportion of grants specifically for health research and, since the launch of the National Institute of Health Research (NIHR) in April 2006 and the implementation of reforms outlined in Best Research for Best Health [1], there has been a strong emphasis on supporting leading research for the benefit of the patient and the public. The creation of this health research system has been endorsed further by the Cooksey report [2], which recognises the role of the NHS in supporting clinical and applied research. These reforms are welcomed as the NIHR's remit for research support includes vital health service and public health research.

The Research for Patient Benefit (RfPB) programme supports research throughout the UK. In 2006, it had an annual budget of approximately £25 million and it consists of ten regional panels that commission local health service research. This programme aims not only to support innovation and developments in healthcare but also to encourage studies related to practice that are identified by NHS staff. It differs from the traditional funding mechanisms, in that it expects the research to be based in an NHS setting and is concerned with the direct impact that the research may have on future practice. The programme also welcomes applications that involve collaboration between the NHS and local universities, thereby encouraging the development of links between primary care and academia.

The bridging of research between the NHS, universities and industry is also supported by Clinical Research Networks (CRNs) across the country. The CRNs are dedicated to supporting everyone involved with research and there are a number of topic-specific networks, as well as those for primary care research and a non-specific Comprehensive Research Network. These networks offer research support to individual researchers and to research groups. They often involve research consultations and training courses that give members access to free expert advice throughout the development of a research project. They are not a source of research grants as such, but they can give advice on grant applications. They can also provide help with patient recruitment once a study is funded and can provide research infrastructure, through Support for Science funding.

As CRNs are in contact with multiple research groups and clinics in a local area, they are also useful in forging collaborations between research groups. Additionally, they provide training sessions on how to apply for funding and will have the most up-to-date information about research funding organisations. As there are so many funding organisations, deciding which one to target can be a daunting task. Therefore, consulting a local CRN about sources of funding available for specific projects is recommended.

Although the internet makes searching for funding a little easier, there are many organisations that support only specific types of research. The coordination of these organisations would be helpful to researchers. To this end, the UK Clinical Research Collaboration (UKCRC) has been set up to provide a forum to facilitate such coordination between funding bodies in specific areas in order to maximise opportunities in health research in the UK.

It is currently mapping a profile of health research being conducted in the UK with the aim of informing the direction for funding in the future. A recent draft report of the UKCRC Sub Committee for Nurses in Clinical Research [3] states that the UKCRC will be allocating some funds to support masters, doctorate, post-doctorate and senior investigator research. This consultation refers to the nursing profession in particular; however it is expected that this will be expanded to include AHPs or a separate AHP scheme may be introduced.

Applying for funding

Applying for funding

Once you have made a confident decision about which organisation to target for funding, the next stage is to write a grant application. Competition for grants being as fierce as it is, only high-quality research proposals, written with precision and clarity, will be considered for funding. The decision to award a grant is made by an expert review panel. The reviewers evaluate all grant applications according to predetermined criteria. These criteria are often given to applicants, with guidelines, and are unique to each funding organisation.

Returning to the internet as a source of information, it is always worth visiting funding bodies' websites to get a feel for which organisation would be suitable for your project. These websites often provide annual reports which describe the projects that they are currently funding. Due to the dynamic nature of health research, funding bodies tend to shift their research interests. You need to make sure that you are up-to-date with current trends. The website for RDFunding (www.rdfunding.org.uk) has an extensive list of links and portals to national and international funding organisations. A list of other useful websites is provided at the end of this chapter.

A good proposal stems from a research idea that makes the reviewers think: 'Yes, of course! Why didn't I think of that?' A project proposal needs to be detailed enough for the readers to understand exactly what the study hopes to achieve and why. It is important to describe clearly the questions which the project will aim to answer and to show that the project is being conducted by investigators with the necessary expertise to achieve the objectives described.

The process of writing the application will often help you to identify what activities, instruments and collaborations are required for the success of the study. These points should be included in the application and will aid in the development of a robust study protocol. The reporting of any preparatory work in the field will always add strength to the application. This demonstrates good planning and commitment to the project, thereby increasing the potential for success. Sorting out this information at the beginning will help clear thinking and organisation of the project.

Writing the proposal

Writing the proposal

The introduction

Although the reviewers may have general expertise and knowledge of research methods, they may not be familiar with the specific proposal area. Therefore, the introduction should describe the context within which the research is to take place. It should demonstrate imaginatively, but logically, that there is a gap in the knowledge and explain how the study will contribute towards filling that gap. A clear definition of the research question, any hypotheses that will be tested and a clear description of the aims and objectives will help to achieve this.

The methods section

This section must be explicit in describing precisely how the study will be conducted. Skill and judgement is required to know what to include as all application forms have a word limit. If well-known methods are going to be used, a single reference is sufficient in place of a full description of the method design, but not if relatively new methods are used. If volunteers are to be used, recruitment policies and inclusion and exclusion criteria must be given. You must also provide a brief description of the evaluation process and your plans for dissemination of the results.

Successful applications are usually composed of a well-defined problem followed by a clear yet simply stated method which demonstrates that the author has not only defined a valid question but also knows how to investigate it. Detail and referencing are important throughout the grant application. No changes can be made to the protocol after acceptance by the grant review panel.

The costs section

The cost of a project must be realistic and allow for the timely completion of the project. There are additional expenses, other than equipment, such as: staff salaries (including pensions and national insurance); pay increases; administration assistance; stationery; and attendance at conferences and meetings. Every item, no matter how small, should be included here as it will not be possible to add to this later. Some institutions may also require you to include an element for overheads. This needs to be established in discussion with the relevant finance officer, according to the institution's policy if the grant-awarding body specifically excludes such overheads (as some do).

The first decision that needs to be made by the chief researcher is whether or not the project will be conducted as part of his or her daily employment. Being a part-time researcher in a clinical post can be a challenging situation to manage. Careful consideration might be needed as to whether the project should be carried out on a full-time basis. If so, it may be useful to look for grants that will provide a full salary for the duration of the proposed project.

If specific equipment is needed for the project, you need to consider its availability within the institute in which the study will be based. Any equipment that needs to be purchased or hired should be included in the costs section of the application. If the study is to be conducted across multiple sites, travel costs should be included. Putting forward collaborative research proposals between researchers in different institutions is an excellent way of increasing the chances of getting funding, particularly if the collaborators are carefully selected for their complementary areas of expertise and include people with an established research reputation.

The curriculum vitae (CV)

The CV will give information about the researchers involved and should include a list of academic publications. This will show whether your team is capable of carrying out the proposed research project. If there is an obvious lack of experience, providing details of collaborators with the relevant knowledge and experience is essential. Without this evidence it is likely that the proposal will be rejected.

Internal scrutiny

The process of writing a grant application is a time-consuming one. You must be able to view the application from all angles and attempt to critique the proposal as the reviewers would. If the criteria for the funding bid are available, the content of the proposal must match that of the funding organisation's requirements. Once the application is complete it is a valuable exercise to subject it to internal scrutiny or peer review before it is sent to external reviewers. If the application is not successful the time will not necessarily have been wasted as the core information can be used for other funding applications.

Questions frequently asked by grant review panels

When writing an application for a grant it is always helpful to consider the types of questions that a review panel might ask. Table 7.1 (below) gives examples of the broad range of questions that may be asked.

Table 7.1

Questions that a grant application should address

Questions that a grant application should address

Is the research proposed important?

- What is the research question?
- Does this fill a gap in knowledge?
- How important is the proposed study to advancing knowledge and understanding in clinical practice?
- Does it address the key challenges in the profession?
- Who will be the target audience for the results?

Can the research be done?

- Are the concepts realistic?
- Are the aims realistic?
- What equipment will be needed?
- Who is involved with the study?
- Is the researcher capable of carrying out the work?
- Can it be done in the specified time?

Are the costs realistic?

- What type of costs will be involved?

What are the broader impacts of the research project?

- How well does the project enhance discovery and understanding?
- What will be the potential benefit of this project to society?
- How will the results be disseminated to the target audience?
- Will the results of the project be useful in institutions other than the one where the study has been conducted?
- Does the project have the potential to lead to the development of a product that will have commercial value?
- Are the plans for developing and distributing any products appropriate and pragmatic?

Conclusion

The process of applying for a research grant involves time and careful planning. A collaborative bid, which includes researchers with the appropriate range of expertise and experience, is often the best route, but this requires considerable prior planning and discussion.

Before attempting to write a proposal, you should research the potential funders and target your application to ensure that your proposed research matches the aims of the funder as closely as possible. The grant application must be clear and concise, describing how the outcomes of the research will add to the existing body of knowledge and benefit the community. This process will help to put the project into perspective and will provide a realistic view of the time and costs involved.

A guide to research for podiatrists

The internal peer review process will ultimately help to refine the proposal in preparation for submission to the chosen funding body. It is always helpful to discuss your ideas with colleagues and seek expert opinion when necessary in order to be confident about the appropriateness of your plans.

References

[1] Department of Health. Best Research for Best Health (London: DH, 2006).

[2] D. Cooksey. A Review of UK Health Research Funding (London: TSO, 2006).

[3] UKCRC Sub Committee for Nurses in Clinical Research (Workforce). *Developing the Best Research Professionals – Qualified Graduate Nurses: Recommendations for preparing and supporting clinical academic nurses of the future*, draft report (London: NHS, 2006).

Useful websites

Best Research for Best Health: A new national health research strategy. Available at www.dh.gov.uk

Department of Trade and Industry. www.dti.gov.uk

Higher Education and Research Opportunities. www.hero.ac.uk

Medical Research Council. www.mrc.ac.uk

National Institute for Health Research. www.nihr.ac.uk

RDFunding. www.rdfunding.org.uk

ResearchResearch. www.researchresearch.com

The Wellcome Trust. www.wellcome.ac.uk

The NHS Health Technology Assessment Programme. www.hta.nhsweb.nhs.uk

UK Clinical Research Network. www.ukcrn.org.uk

Chapter 8
Obtaining ethical approval

Jackie Campbell and Mike Curran

Ethical practice in research is as important as ethical clinical practice and history has shown that it cannot be left to chance. Clinical practice focuses on the best interests of the individual as an inherent part of the process, but often research is conducted on one group for the benefit of others. Decisions have to be made as to whether the disadvantages for the few are balanced by the advantages for the many. Researchers themselves are often not the best people to judge this and there have been some bad mistakes in the past, most driven by the incentive to do good science.

The recent Alder Hey retained organs scandal is just one example [1]. As a result of past mistakes, and the resultant public outcry, increased regulation has been introduced for research which involves the NHS and puts a statutory requirement on researchers to gain approval from a formally constituted research ethics committee before their research can be undertaken. Similar systems are in place for research within social services.

This has also had knock-on effects for research outside these services as the threshold for demonstrating ethical practice of research has been raised. Those undertaking research in areas not covered by the regulations also now need to show that an equivalent level of scrutiny has taken place or run the risk of litigation if complaints are made.

What needs formal approval?

The Research Governance Framework

Formal approval

The Research Governance Framework [2] states that the dignity, rights, safety and well-being of participants must be the primary consideration of any research study and sets out the requirements for approval of research carried out under the auspices of the

NHS. Those requirements and the associated procedures are slightly different for the four home nations, but the principles are the same. (See 'Further information' at the end of this chapter for details of where to find full documentation.) Research involving any of the following must receive ethical approval from a Research Ethics Committee (REC) constituted for that purpose by the Department of Health (or its other national counterparts):

- patients and users of the NHS – includes all participants recruited by virtue of their past or present treatment by, or use of, the NHS and includes NHS patients treated under contract by the private sector;
- participants recruited because they are relatives or carers of the above;
- access to data, organs or other bodily material of past or present NHS patients –includes the retrospective use of patient records;
- fetal material and IVF involving NHS patients;
- the recently dead in NHS premises;
- the use of, or potential access to, NHS premises or facilities;
- NHS staff – recruited as research participants by virtue of their professional role.

This is a very wide-ranging list. In summary, any research that involves NHS patients, staff or premises must go through the formal REC approval process. These processes have been the subject of recent review, the results of which are currently being implemented (see 'Future developments', p. 68). For up-to-date information consult your Trust's R&D lead or the National Research Ethics Service (previously known as the Central Office for Research Ethics Committees (COREC) and now part of the National Patient Safety Agency) who have a good website, full of the appropriate forms and guidance notes (www.nres.npsa.nhs.uk).

Research, clinical audit or service evaluation?

What is research?

The Research Governance Framework only covers activity that is defined as research. This begs many questions and provokes many arguments as people, understandably, try to cut down on the bureaucracy by avoiding the REC approval process. Table 8.1 (opposite) explains the current definitions [3].

Table 8.1

Differentiating research, audit and evaluation

Differentiating research, audit and evaluation

Research	Clinical audit	Service evaluation
Designed and conducted to generate new knowledge	Designed and conducted to provide new knowledge to provide best care	Designed and conducted to define current care
Quantitative research – hypothesis based Qualitative research – explores themes following established methodology	Designed to answer the question: 'Does this service reach a predetermined standard?'	Designed to answer the question: 'What standard does this service reach?'
	Measures against a standard	Measures current service without reference to a standard
May involve a new treatment	Does not involve a new treatment	Does not involve a new treatment
May involve additional therapies, samples or investigations	Involves no more than administration of questionnaire or record analysis	Involves no more than administration of simple interview, questionnaire or record analysis
May involve allocation to treatment groups not chosen by the health professional responsible for care or patient	Does not involve allocation to treatment groups: the health professional responsible for care and patients chooses treatment	Does not involve allocation to treatment groups: the health professional responsible for care and patients chooses treatment
May involve randomisation	Does not involve randomisation	Does not involve randomisation

Although any of these may raise ethical issues, under current guidance:

Research requires REC review	Clinical audit does not require REC review	Service evaluation does not require REC review

Whilst it may seem attractive to redefine your research question in terms of clinical audit or evaluation, there are drawbacks. Firstly, you may not be able to publish your results in a research journal. Most require evidence of REC approval before they will publish. Secondly, even though you may not need to submit the

REC paperwork, you will almost certainly have to get approval from the Trust under its procedures for the audit or evaluation. The Trust also will not be able to count your project towards its annual reporting of research activity, which could affect its future research funding. Take advice before you decide how to categorise your work.

Future developments

Future developments

Research involving only NHS staff as participants has been particularly problematic for researchers, especially those undertaking small, local projects as it has meant that even interviewing one member of NHS staff, or circulating a questionnaire to staff in a department, has involved a full REC application. Also, the situation regarding the use of anonymised patient data has been confused.

There has been a review of the NHS research ethics procedures (the Warner report [4]) and a consultation has been undertaken with a view to streamlining the processes and redefining the categories of research which are required to go through full review. The response to the consultation [5] chose not to redefine the categories but has recommended that a lighter touch process may be introduced for 'low-risk' research projects. A new independent group of National Research Ethics Advisers has been proposed which will perform a screening function on applications to identify applications which:

- fall outside the remit of NHS RECs;
- are of poor quality;
- apparently present no material ethical issues;
- or are complex or involve unfamiliar research methods.

Those studies which present few ethical issues will be considered by a streamlined process of review by a small executive group, whereas more complex studies will go to full committee and may require additional expert opinion.

All NHS research will still need to get local Trust approval from the R&D department and they will guide you as to what the current requirements are.

What does NHS ethical approval involve?

Ethical approval

You will not be able to apply for ethical approval until the planning for your project is at a highly advanced stage. The REC will need a detailed picture of your research: why it is needed, who the participants will be, what information they will be given, what resources are required, where it will be done, by whom it will be done and, most importantly, a detailed protocol giving as much information as possible about the methods to be used and the mechanics of how the project will be undertaken.

RECs are organised by 'domains'. A domain is defined as a Strategic Health Authority (England), a Health Board (Scotland), a Regional Office of the NHS Wales Department or the whole of Northern Ireland. If your research will be carried out at just one Trust, or several Trusts within the same domain, then you contact your local REC coordinator and arrange for it to be considered by one of the committees within that domain. However, if you are involving Trusts across more than one domain, then it has to go to a committee authorised to deal with multi-site applications (a multi-site REC, or MREC).

There is a telephone booking system for these applications. Details of how to apply and the online forms which need to be completed, are available from the COREC website (www.nres.npsa.nhs.uk). Table 8.2 (overleaf) reproduces the document checklist which has to accompany each application [6]. This table applies to non-drug trials (formally referred to as clinical trials of investigational medicinal products or CTIMPs) as these have additional requirements. Not all the items are required for each project, as the system has to take into account a very wide range of possible types of research project. However, you have to complete the form and provide a protocol and investigator's CV and will usually have to include at least a participant information sheet and consent form. There are guidelines to follow for the production of all of these on the COREC site.

You will probably be invited to attend the committee meeting. If at all possible, do try to go. It can be daunting (you can take someone with you for support) but it can help, as you can probably answer most of the committee's queries on the spot. They will issue their decision in writing soon after the meeting. They may be able to give an immediate 'favourable opinion' (approval) or they may need further clarification or amendments.

A guide to research for podiatrists

Table 8.2   **Applicant checklist for Research Ethics Committee**

Document	Enclosed?	Date	Version	Office use
Covering letter on headed paper	Yes / No			
NHS REC Application Form, Parts A&B	Mandatory			
Site-Specific Information Form (for SSA)	Yes / No			
Research protocol (6 copies) or project proposal	Mandatory			
Summary CV for Chief Investigator (CI)	Mandatory			
Summary CV for supervisor (student research)	Yes / No			
Research participant information sheet (PIS)	Yes / No			
Research participant consent form	Yes / No			
Letters of invitation to participants	Yes / No			
GP/Consultant information sheets or letters	Yes / No			
Statement of indemnity arrangements	Yes / No			
Letter from sponsor	Yes / No			
Letter from statistician	Yes / No			
Letter from funder	Yes / No			
Referees' or other scientific critique report	Yes / No			
Summary, synopsis or diagram (flowchart) of protocol in non-technical language	Yes / No			
Interview schedules or topic guides for participants	Yes / No			
Validated questionnaire	Yes / No			
Non-validated questionnaire	Yes / No			
Copies of advertisement material for research participants, e.g. posters, newspaper adverts, website. For video or audio cassettes, please also provide the printed script.	Yes / No			

This is not the end! Each project also has to have local R&D management approval and some may need Site Specific Approval. If you are not an employee of the Trust you may need to have an honorary research contract and some Trusts require their researchers to have completed a training course which complies with the International Conference on Harmonisation – Good Clinical Practice (ICH GCP) guidelines [7]. At the moment, each Trust has its own procedure for all this, although the forms are now common (on the National Research Ethics Service website). You need to discuss this with your R&D lead. You may sometimes be able to carry out these processes in parallel but you cannot proceed with the research until everything has been approved.

All this takes a lot of time. When planning your project, you should allow at least six months to produce the documentation and get the necessary approvals.

Non-NHS research

Non-NHS research

All of the above is a requirement of the Research Governance Frameworks. Strictly speaking, it is not required for non-NHS research. However, this Framework has set the standard and the expectations will be that all research should meet it. All universities now have their own research ethics committees which consider non-NHS research to which staff and students must submit their projects for approval.

Research which is undertaken on patients in private practice, for whom no NHS payments are made, is not required to go through REC approval. In theory, a researcher can just do it. However, they may find that they are unable to publish the results without evidence of an independent ethical review. Also, increasing litigation may mean that a research participant could sue for harm or negligence and, without evidence that the research adhered to at least the same standards as those in the NHS, the researcher would probably not have a defence. NHS RECs are open to anyone to submit research projects to, and, for larger projects, it may be sensible to do this. For small projects, you should at least seek some external review of the ethical issues, and have this documented.

What are the main ethical issues?

Ethical issues

In practical terms, the following are the main issues that you need to consider in the design of your research. Your solutions to them will need to be made explicit in any application for ethical approval.

Informed consent

- What information will be given to participants in writing? Is the style appropriate to your participants? Will the participants get an opportunity to discuss it as well as read it?
- It must be made explicit that there will be no penalty for those who refuse to participate or who drop out.
- Is there a power relationship between the person obtaining the consent and the participant (for example, a manager researching their own staff or a healthcare practitioner and their own patients)? If so, there could be implied coercion to participate.
- Good practice requires an opt-in system (patients make a conscious decision to take part).
- Will participants get paid? Good practice encourages extra expenses (such as travel) to be reimbursed but not at a level sufficient to be an incentive.
- Are participants from a vulnerable group (for example, children or cognitively impaired)? If so, what special arrangements are being made for consent. (This is a complex legal area and special arrangements for others to consent or give assent on their behalf maybe possible. You need to seek advice.)
- Are you unnecessarily excluding some participants because of practical difficulties (for example, vulnerable groups or those who are not fluent in English)? If so, you may be excluding these populations from the benefits of research findings.
- Will you be audio- or video-taping the participants? If so, it is good practice to obtain specific consent for this.

Confidentiality

Identifying information should be removed as soon as possible in the research process and be replaced with a coded identifier if it may be necessary for the researcher (and only the researcher) to trace information back at a later stage. The code should be kept securely. Codes such as initials or dates of birth do not protect confidentiality.

Care should be taken when reporting findings so that the identity of participants cannot be inferred. This is particularly important in qualitative research and when quantitative results are divided down into very small subsets.

Data should be held securely in locked filing cabinets and password-protected PCs. It is good practice not to hold identifiable data on computers outside the workplace.

Potential harm

In the worst case, what possible physical harm might arise from this research and what steps are being taken to prevent or mitigate this?

Could participants suffer mental distress as a result of this research? Does the project explore potentially distressing issues or ones that could cause the participants to become upset? If so, what arrangements are being made for counselling and the like?

Will the participants be inconvenienced (for example, by having to attend extra clinics or have additional blood samples taken)? If so, have they been fully informed?

Is there potential danger to the researcher? If the researcher will be making domiciliary visits, what arrangements have been made to ensure his or her safety?

What insurance or indemnity arrangements are in place in case of a claim of negligent harm? Are there arrangements for non-negligent harm? There are not usually such arrangements, which is acceptable as long as that is made explicit.

Methodology

Has the protocol been independently reviewed? Bad research is unethical as it, at best, inconveniences participants with no prospect of answering the research question or, at worst, leads to misleading findings becoming disseminated.

For quantitative studies, has the project had documented advice from an independent statistician? This is essential to ensure, for example, that the sample size is sufficient to show the intended outcome.

For randomised trials, is there a control or placebo arm? Although this can be the best research design, it can be unethical if it deprives patients of the current best treatment. Randomised trials should compare the test treatment with the standard current treatment.

Conflict of interest

For instance, has the study been funded by a body which may have an interest in a particular outcome?

Conclusion

Research ethics are complex and some issues that need to be considered may not be obvious at first sight. The procedures involved in getting ethical approval are also complex and require much time and effort. These processes are often cited as the reason for not carrying out research, particularly small-scale projects. However, there is nothing in the ethical approval process that should not have been thought about and documented as part of the normal research process.

All research projects should have a detailed protocol; all should respect the rights and dignity of the participants; all participants should have written information about the project and so on. The research ethics approval process forces researchers to do this at the point when it needs to be done – before the project starts. There have been problems with the NHS procedures but these are now bedding down and there are plans to streamline them further.

There is therefore no reason for your project not to undergo full ethical approval, and the potential dangers of not doing so should provide an added incentive. You should take advice early on in the research planning process – from your Trust R&D department (for NHS staff) or from the local Research & Development Support Unit (see Further information, p.75).

References

[1] M. Redfern, J. Keeling and E. Powell. *The Report of the Royal Liverpool Children's Hospital Inquiry* (London: TSO, 2001).

[2] Department of Health. Research governance framework for health and social care, 2nd edn (London: DH, 2005).

[3] COREC Ethics Consultation e-Group. *Differentiating audit, service evaluation and research*. Available at www.nres.npsa.nhs.uk. Accessed 2.6.06.

[4] Department of Health. *Report of the Ad Hoc Advisory Group on the Operation of NHS Research Ethics Committees* (London: DH, 2005).

[5] COREC. *Building on improvement: Implementing the recommendations of the Report of the Ad Hoc Advisory Group on the Operation of NHS Research Ethics Committees*. Available at www.nres.npsa.nhs.uk. Accessed 5.3.07.

[6] COREC. *Applicant's checklist*. Available at www.nres.npsa.nhs.uk. Accessed 13.6.07.

[7] European Medicines Agency. *ICH Topic E6 (R1) Guidelines for Good Clinical Practice*. Available at www.emea.europa.eu. Accessed 5.3.07.

Further information

National Research Ethics Service. www.nres.npsa.nhs.uk

Research Governance Framework (links to framework documents for England, Scotland, Waltes and Northern Ireland). Available at: www.dh.gov.uk

Chapter on Research Ethics from the World Medical Assembly Medical Ethics manual. Available at www.wma.net

RCN Handbook on Research Ethics: Guidance for nurses (London: RCN, 2007)

List of Research and Development Support Units. Available at: www.trentrdsu.org.uk

Chapter 9
Numerical data analysis

Jackie Campbell and Farina Hashmi

There is something about numbers – you either love them or loathe them. Numerical data is a critical source of evidence and can be extremely powerful, with the right treatment. But, as in many other specialisms, the impenetrable jargon and arcane procedures of statistics can put off all but the most dedicated.

This chapter does not set out to teach numerical analysis, but introduces some of the main topics to give a basis on which to build with more detailed reading elsewhere. It will set out the principles behind numerical data and its analysis and enable you to begin to understand the basic analysis described in research papers and discuss your own research needs with a statistician. A guide to where to find further information can be found at the end of the chapter.

Statistics

Statistics

Statistics provide researchers and scientists with a way of describing and understanding the world through mathematics. They help us to make sense of the decisions we need to make in our daily professional activities. In the health sciences, statistics often allow numbers relating to a population to be estimated when the whole population cannot be directly studied due to practicalities or restrictions in time, money, or other resources.

The research journey begins at the planning stage, which leads to the design of the project. It is at this stage that the types of data that you will be working with, the questions that you want to ask of the data, the way that the data will be sampled and collected and the appropriate analytical tools to answer those questions must be considered. If you ignore these issues at this point you may find that you have not collected the appropriate data for your project. It is

A guide to research for podiatrists

essential to seek advice from a statistician at an early stage. You can get statistical advice from most NHS Trust R&D departments and R&D Support Units (see 'Further information', p.85) and universities. Feedback at this stage is invaluable in developing a well-designed project. You will also need statistical advice later on, when analysing the data and interpreting the results.

It is important to understand the central role of statistics in scientific health research. We need to understand the scope of the statistical tests used; what the common types of data are; the distribution of that data and the concepts of error and random variation. There are two categories of statistics: descriptive and inferential statistics.

Descriptive statistics

Descriptive statistics

Descriptive statistics provide tools to describe data and are often an ideal point to start when trying to make sense of data that has been collected. This process allows the researcher to get a feel for the data and to describe the characteristics of the sample population. Sometimes this is all that is needed – for example, if you just want to report the percentage of staff working part-time or the success rate of a procedure in your own department.

Most often, the data that has been collected will need to be summarised in a digestible form. To do this, we need to quote a 'typical' or average value but, to give a fuller picture of the data, we also need to convey how variable the data is. To do this, we need measures of spread.

Averages (or 'measures of central tendency')

There are three 'averages', each suited to different situations. It is common for the wrong average to be quoted when people are trying to put over a point, for example when quoting 'average' salaries as part of pay negotiations. This can be very confusing and the word 'average' is best avoided altogether.

The **mean** is calculated by adding together all the numbers in a data set and dividing the total by the number of separate scores. So, from the following set of scores: 12, 40, 20, 10, the mean of these four scores would be $82 \div 4 = 20.5$. This value is only meaningful when it describes a set of data which is roughly symmetrical – that is, where the high values are balanced by low ones. It is very prone to distortion by a few very high (or very low) values (for instance, in the example of pay negotiations, the chief executive's salary).

The **median** is the middle value from a set of scores and represents the central point in a data set which has been put into size, or rank, order. For example, from five bars of chocolate weighing 20, 40, 60, 100 and 200 grams each, the median value would be 60. This is a useful measure when the data is not distributed symmetrically (a skewed distribution) because, as the median is determined by its position in the ranked list, not by the values of the other points, it is not affected by extreme points. Half of the data points will be less than (or equal to) the median, and half will be greater than (or equal to) it.

The **mode** is the most commonly occurring value in a data set. Therefore, from the following: 5, 6, 7, 8, 9, 9, 9, 9, 9, 10 the number 9 would be the value occurring most often. This has limited applications but can be useful if you want to record the most frequently occurring value. There may be more than one mode in a data set (for example, the set 5, 6, 6, 6, 7, 8, 9, 9, 9, 10 has modal values of 6 and 9).

Measures of spread

The **standard deviation** is a measure of spread of the data on either side of the mean and is used when the data is symmetrical. For this sort of data, the mean and standard deviation tend to be quoted together to give a summary of the data.

When the data is not symmetrical, the median is used as the average (see above). The concept of the halfway point can be extended to define the two points which represent the quarter and three-quarter points in a ranked list. These values are called the **inter-quartile range**. In total, 50 per cent of the data points will lie between the two values defined by the inter-quartile range (and 25 per cent will be less than or equal to the lower value and 25 per cent greater than or equal to the upper value).

Figure 9.1 (overleaf) shows an example of the three types of average calculated for a set of data on the length of time that patients having a particular operation stay in hospital (a skewed distribution). It also shows the inter-quartile range – 50 per cent of the patients stay between four and seven days.

Figure 9.1

A skewed distribution, showing mean, median, mode and interquartile range

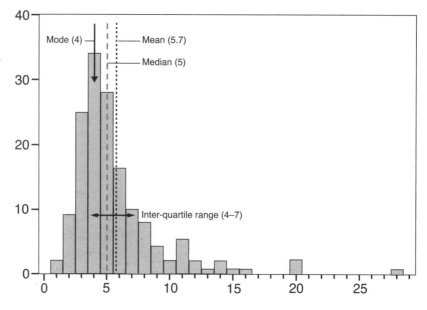

Inferential statistics

Inferential statistics use information from a sample in order to make inferences about the population from which the sample was drawn. These tests are important in ensuring that the results from the sample are generalisable to the wider population, given the evidence provided by the research. Such analysis enables the researcher to make predictions from the data and test a hypothesis. The big assumption that is being made for all of these tests is that the research design was flawless. In particular, they assume that the data was collected from a truly random sample from the larger population of interest.

Statistical tests

Statistical tests

The most common statistical tests are those that compare groups of data for differences or for relationships. The choice of which test to use depends on:

- what question is being asked;
- the type of data used;
- whether the data is 'Normally distributed';
- the size of the samples;
- the number of sample groups;

- whether data was collected under different conditions from the same group (paired data) or from different groups (independent samples).

Types of data

Nominal data includes data such as yes or no answers, ethnicity or eye colour. There is no rank order to this type of data. You couldn't say that 'blue eyes' were greater than 'brown eyes'. Categories can, of course, be coded by assigning numbers. This is often done to aid computer analysis of this type of data. However, just because a category or value is represented by a number does not make the data numerical. For example, in the International Classification of Diseases (ICD) [1], onycholysis is coded as L60.1 whilst onychogryphosis is L60.2. This obviously doesn't mean that onychgryphosis is somehow 'bigger' than onycholysis.

Ordinal data, by contrast, is data that can be put into an ordered, or ranked, list. The Likert Scale is an example of this and is often used in questionnaires. Patient satisfaction questionnaires often use this design, where the scale ranges from 'very unsatisfied' to 'very satisfied'. Other options run in order between these two endpoints such as 'unsatisfied', 'unsure' and 'satisfied'. Again, there are no meaningful measurements between these options but they form an order of preference. However, the sizes of the differences between each item on the list are not necessarily the same. For example, the difference between unsatisfied and unsure may not be equal to that between satisfied and very satisfied.

Interval data is data that has meaningful spaces between the measurements such as temperature (in degrees) or length (in mm). With interval data, the distances between the values on a scale have meaning. If we use temperature for example, the difference between 40°C and 80°C is the same as the difference between 60°C and 100°C.

Ratio data also has a rank order and equal differences between the values representing equal changes in the measured quantity (as for interval data). The additional requirement is that multiples (or fractions) are also meaningful. For example, 4 kg is twice as heavy as 2 kg, or 40 ml is one quarter the volume of 160 ml.

A guide to research for podiatrists

Normal distributions

The Normal distribution is the name given to a special type of symmetrical distribution which has unique mathematical properties that can be used to make statistical predictions. The name is confusing and does not imply absence of abnormality. It is often referred to by the shape of the histogram that the data produces – the 'bell-shaped curve' – or sometimes as the Gaussian distribution. Much of the data relating to human, animal and plant characteristics is Normally distributed.

Figure 9.2 shows an example of a Normal distribution. This is a histogram of the heights of 151 older women in half-centimetre intervals [2]. This sample had a mean height of 159.8 cm and a standard deviation of 6.03 cm. As it is a fairly small sample, the histogram looks a bit 'blocky', but it is obviously higher in the middle, lower at both sides and is more or less symmetrical. If a huge sample were taken so that the height intervals on the histogram could be very narrow, then the smooth curve shown would represent a line joining the tops of all the columns. This line is the theoretical Normal curve.

Figure 9.2

A Normal distribution

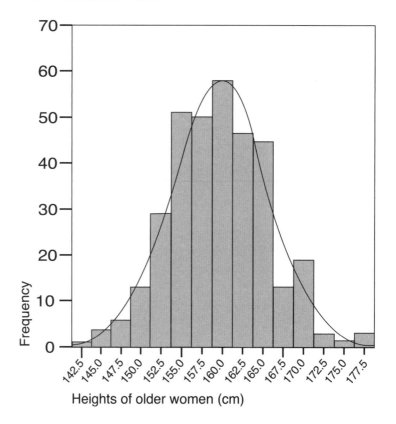

Numerical data analysis

There are essentially two groups of statistical tests: parametric and non-parametric. The former applies to data that has a Normal distribution, the latter makes no assumptions about the shape of the distribution.

Parametric tests are more powerful than their non-parametric counterparts in that they find differences or associations (where they really exist) with smaller sample sizes. However, using these tests inappropriately will produce misleading results. For parametric tests, data should conform to the following conditions:

- be interval or ratio data;

- have a Normal distribution;

- have a sample size of at least 30.

Figure 9.3 (below) shows a simple flow chart for determining which of the most common tests should be used for which situation.

Figure 9.3

Flowchart for selecting statistical tests

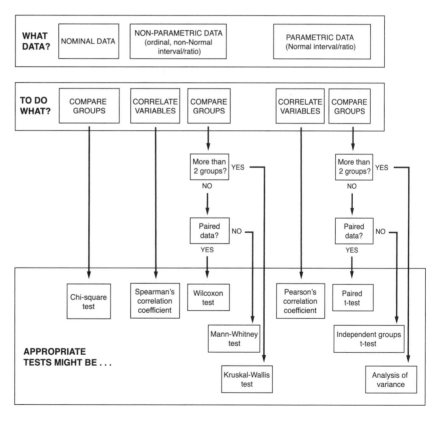

Interpreting the results of statistical tests

The main output from a statistical test is the value of a test statistic (specific to the test being performed), calculated from the data, and an associated p value: p here stands for probability, or likelihood, and is represented by a number from 0 (no chance at all) to 1 (absolute certainty). It is also sometimes represented as a percentage (by multiplying it by a hundred) and may be referred to as the significance level. This figure gives the likelihood of achieving that value for the test statistic purely by chance. (The lower it is, the more likely your results are to be significant.)

For example, a study which looked at the efficacy of a new wound dressing showed that there was a mean healing time which was 3.2 days shorter than when using standard treatment. This study was carried out on a sample of the whole population who might use this dressing. If the study were to be repeated with two other groups with the same sample size, you would not expect the mean difference to be exactly 3.2 days due to the innate variability in people's healing mechanisms. And if you repeated the study many times, you might find that, in some cases, the standard treatment gives quicker healing, or that, averaged out over all the studies, there is no difference (mean difference of zero).

However, using our initial study, we could say that 3.2 days is our best estimate of the mean difference in healing times for the population. The real question is, how big does that difference have to be before we can be confident that it is not just a random variation from a true population mean difference of zero. We might be very confident about saying that it is a real difference if the new treatment cut ten days off the standard healing time. We might be very confident about 3.2 days being a real improvement if we knew that the study had been done with a sample of 5,000 patients. We also might be reassured if we knew that people's healing rates varied very little from person to person in our population of interest.

The statistical test takes into account the size of the difference, the variability of the data and the sample sizes, and calculates how likely it is that a difference of 3.2 days could have arisen purely by chance if the real difference was zero. Let us say that this likelihood was calculated by the statistical test and reported as p = 0.03. There is then a 3 per cent chance that the outcome of the study was just a chance occurrence and not related to the intervention being studied. It therefore seems likely that we are seeing a true difference between the two dressings.

How sure do you want to be?

How sure do you want to be?

There will always be a chance that any result could have been achieved by chance, albeit a very small one in some cases. You have to decide how much of a risk you want to take that the results are just random fluctuation when conluding that your results are positive.

There is a trade-off here. The smaller the risk you are willing to take that you might be wrong in asserting a true difference, or association, in your results, the bigger the risk that you are being unnecessarily cautious (saying there is no difference when there really is). The usual 'benchmark' risk of apparently positive results being due to chance is 5 per cent or p = 0.05. (In other words, if p = 0.05, it would usually be considered reasonable to assert that you have recorded a positive result.) However, there may be good reasons for choosing more or less cautious figures such as 0.01 (1 per cent) or 0.1 (10 per cent) in your own particular circumstances.

References

[1] World Health Organisation. *International Statistical Classification of Diseases and Related Health Problems* (Geneva: WHO, 1994).

[2] D. J. Hand, F. Daly, A. D. Lunn, K. J. McConway and E. Ostrowski. *A Handbook of Small Data Sets* (London: Chapman and Hall, 1994).

Further information

There is a huge number of books on statistics and data analysis. These are just a few, suitable for the non-specialist.

F. Clegg. *Simple Statistics: A course book for the social sciences* (Cambridge: Cambridge University Press, 1990).

S. Polgar and S. A. Thomas. *Introduction to Research in the Health Sciences*, 4th edn (Edinburgh: Elsevier Churchill Livingstone, 2000).

N. Mathers, M. Williams and B. Hancock (eds). *Statistical Analysis in Primary*

Care (Abingdon: Radcliffe Medical Press, 2000).

D. Coggon, *Statistics in Clinical Practice*, 2nd edn (London: BMJ Publishing Group, 2003).

D. Bowers. *Statistics from Scratch: An introduction for health care professionals* (Chichester: Wiley, 1996).

D. Bowers. *Further Statistics from Scratch for Healthcare Professionals* (Chichester: Wiley, 1997).

M. H. Katz. *Study Design and Statistical Analysis: A practical guide for clinicians* (Cambridge: Cambridge University Press, 2006).

C. M. Hicks. *Research for Physiotherapists: Project design and analysis*, 2nd edn (Edinburgh: Churchill Livingstone, 1995).

There is also a useful collection of web-based resources on statistics at www.trentrdsu.org.uk.

For advice on statistics, contact your local NHS Trust R&D department or your local R&D Support Unit (RDSU). You can find details of your nearest RDSU at www.trentrdsu.org.uk.

Chapter 10
Qualitative analysis
Lisa Farndon and Alan Borthwick

Data generated from quantitative studies will usually be numerical, whereas a qualitative study will generate textual data. The text will most commonly be in the form of transcripts of interviews, written observations of situations or other documents and records. Qualitative studies can generate a huge number of words and make analysis a time-consuming process. But it is important, because the aim of that analysis is to identify themes to explain the situation you have chosen to investigate.

You can choose from a number of different methods to analyse your data, but they all involve: organising the data; generating categories; themes and patterns; testing emergent hypotheses against the data; searching for alternative explanations of the data; and writing up the results.

Methods

Methods

One of the most commonly used methods of data analysis is the framework approach [1], which has five stages:

Familiarisation – the data is read a number of times to get an overview of the content

Identifying a thematic framework – key issues, concepts and themes are identified; this may be based on the original research questions

Indexing – the thematic framework is then used to order the data systematically into categories

Charting – charts are devised with headings to represent main themes and sub-headings for minor themes

Mapping and interpretation – the data is sifted and charted according to core themes and analysed in order to define concepts, find associations and provide explanations for the data.

Thematic analysis has also been proposed as a method to identify, analyse and report patterns (themes) within qualitative data [2]. Boyatzis [3] and Ryan and Bernard [4] report that this method can be used to analyse qualitative data generated by different research methods.

Braun and Clarke [2] believe that thematic analysis can be used as an independent research method, regardless of the philosophical stance of the researcher. Its implementation and the findings that are generated should match the initial assumptions of the study and be made explicit to the reader of the final written report. This method should supply a detailed and rich description of the data.

Although most qualitative research techniques adopt a more inductive approach than quantitative methods, Ryan and Bernard [4] view thematic analysis as either coming from an inductive or deductive stance. Themes or patterns may be identified that emerge from the data (inductive) or be deduced based on the original aims of the research and guided by the interview questions asked (deductive).

Pope *et al.* [5] also reiterate this point when discussing the framework approach for analysing data, by stating that a deductive overview is employed based on predetermined aims and objectives, although the themes will still be grounded in the data reflecting participants' accounts.

During the analysis phase of a qualitative study, data or text is processed or reduced by the researcher so it can be more easily manipulated and themes or patterns can be identified. Braun and Clarke [2] describe this as comprising:

- gaining familiarity with the text
- generating initial codes
- searching for themes
- reviewing themes
- defining and naming themes
- and producing a final report.

The analysis phase is said to be complete if no new themes are emerging or being found in the data. This stage is referred to as saturation.

Rigour

Rigour

The quantitative research process aims to reduce or eliminate bias and manipulate the data produced (in the form of numbers) objectively, using statistical tests to show patterns and provide evidence for hypotheses. Qualitative analysis works with words rather than numbers and so different processes have been introduced to try and ensure that rigour is maintained. Five concepts associated with rigour in qualitative work have been described [6]:

Credibility – this is an alternative to validity in quantitative research studies and aims to match what is reported by the researcher to the research question [7]. There are a number of ways to increase the credibility of findings. Some researchers advise sending the results after analysis back to the original participants or people with similar attributes to see whether they agree with the findings.

Dependability – this is an alternative to reliability in quantitative research and should ensure that data collection is consistent. This can be achieved by using a number of different researchers to analyse the same data and then checking that they have all assigned the same category to each excerpt [8].

Confirmability – the researcher should clearly show the processes by which the data was collected, analysed and presented (a decision trail) [9] and make these transparent to ensure that anyone reading the research can understand how decisions about the data were made.

Transferability – this is an exploration of whether the findings of the research could be transferred to other populations and is similar to the concept of generalisability.

Triangulation – this is the use of multiple investigators or different analysis methods to improve the dependability of the findings and reduce bias [7]. This also gives an opportunity to explore negative or deviant cases, which do not fit into a pattern, which should also be reported and explained if possible.

Reflexivity should also play a part in the qualitative research process [10]. This is when researchers state their position and views, as total detachment is impossible and researcher involvement in the whole process is bound to influence the interpretation of the data [11].

Assessing and analysing documents

Analysis of documents requires a further set of robust criteria to ensure validity [12–14]. In research terms, a 'document' can be anything from an official report to a personal diary, letter, photograph or even a gravestone inscription. It might also apply to video film or other related media – any 'persistent entity'. However, for the most part, documents are classified into public records, the media, private papers, biography and visual documents. Why, and for whom, these documents have been constructed is an essential consideration when attempting to analyse their content and understand their meaning. The key criteria by which they are judged are: credibility, authenticity, representativeness and meaning:

Credibility refers to the extent to which the document is sincere and accurate – in other words, how distorted the contents are likely to be. In order to make a judgement, you need to understand the circumstances under which people may be insincere or inaccurate.

Authenticity refers to soundness and authorship – genuineness, whether a document is what it purports to be. Is it an original or a copy or a copy of a copy? Who wrote it and how can you be reasonably sure that they did indeed write it?

Representativeness refers to survival and availability – is the document representative of the totality of relevant documents? If, for instance, you wanted to look at the number of times articles on rheumatoid arthritis were published in the *British Journal of Podiatry*, you would need access to a complete journal collection – missing a year or two would render the result invalid.

Meaning refers to literal and interpretive understanding – from simply being able to read the document (reading hand-written letters can sometimes be a problem, or perhaps documents translated from another language) to understanding the nuances that might require a deep understanding of the context in which it was written (for example, ploughing through a government White Paper requires this sort of skill).

Documents can be analysed thematically, as described above, or by content analysis, which is really a quantitative technique – counting the number of times a phrase or theme occurs.

Software packages

Software packages

A number of computer packages are now available to manage qualitative data and aid in the analysis process to improve rigour. One of the most common is NViVo (www.qsrinternational.com). Although such programs may help to organise data, they are still time-consuming to use and the researcher will still need to deduce theory or explanations based on the themes derived from the data.

Presentation of data

Presentation of data

When writing up interview-based research, you need to provide a narrative along with the presuppositions of the researcher and the process by which these merged during the analysis. This is sometimes referred to as a decision trail. This should allow the reader to evaluate the quality of the research [15].

However, the social contexts of the participants' experiences should also be considered during interpretation, along with reflection on the personal experiences of the researcher to show how views and interpretations expressed in the work were shaped. You should also include descriptions of occasions where the interpretations of the researcher and participants vary to show the open nature of the interpretation, how the themes were derived and the interpretive framework used.

Using direct data extracts from interview transcripts is an integral part of the data presentation. These give the reader an insight into the actual words spoken by the interviewees and allow a judgment to be made about the author's interpretation of the data presented. They are usually identified in the text by italicisation and the use of single line spacing, where the rest of the text is 1.5 or double-spaced. The supporting narrative provides a background context which should help the reader appreciate the meaning by understanding a little of the social environment in which the interviewee is embedded.

A guide to research for podiatrists

References

[1]   J. Ritchie and L. Spencer. Qualitative data analysis for applied policy research. In *Analysing Qualitative Data*, eds A. Bryman and R.G. Burgess (London: Routledge, 1994).

[2]   V. Braun and V. Clarke. Using thematic analysis in psychology. *Qualitative Research in Psychology*, 3 (2006), 77–101.

[3]   R.E. Boyatzis. *Transforming Qualitative Information: Thematic analysis and code development* (Thousand Oaks, CA: Sage, 1998).

[4]   G. W. Ryan and H. R. Bernard. Data management and analysis methods. In *Handbook of Qualitative Research*, 2nd edn, eds N. K. Denzin and Y. S. Lincoln (Thousand Oaks, CA: Sage, 2000).

[5]   C. Pope, S. Ziebland and N. Mays. Qualitative Research in Health Care: Analysing qualitative data. *British Medical Journal*, 320 (2000), 114–6.

[6]   E. G. Guba and Y. S. Lincoln. Competing paradigms in qualitative research. In *Handbook of Qualitative Research*, eds N. K. Denzin and Y. S. Lincoln (Thousand Oaks, CA: Sage, 1994).

[7]   T. Long and M. Johnson. Rigour, reliability and validity in qualitative research. *Clinical Effectiveness in Nursing*, 4 (2000), 30–7.

[8]   M. Hammersley. The generalisability of ethnography. In *What's Wrong with Ethnography?*, ed. M. Hammersley (London: Routledge, 1992).

[9]   J. Popay, A. Rogers and G. Williams. Rationale and standards for the systematic review of qualitative literature in health services research. *Qualitative Health Research*, 8 (1998), 341–51.

[10] D. Horsburgh. Evaluation of qualitative research. *Journal of Clinical Nursing*, 12 (2003), 307–12.

[11] J. Mason. *Qualitative Researching* (London: Sage, 1996).

[12] K. Macdonald. Using documents. In *Researching Social Life*, ed. N. Gilbert (London: Sage, 2001).

[13] J. Scott. *A Matter of Record: Documentary sources in social research* (Cambridge: Polity Press, 1990).

[14] K. Plummer. *Documents of life* (London: Unwin Hyman, 1983).

[15] C. B. Draucker. The critique of Heideggerian hermeneutic nursing research. *Journal of Advanced Nursing*, 30 (1999), 60–73.

Chapter 11
Disseminating research findings
Andrew Barnes and Mike Curran

This chapter is for anyone who might be considering how to convey the results of their research to an audience. Whilst it is not an exhaustive article and not intended as a complete guide, the aim is to communicate our personal views and advice on some aspects of research dissemination.

We have focused on the two most common forms of communicating research findings – written and audio-visual presentation. Other related issues are also touched on, such as the motivations for communicating, the forums that can be used, when these forums might be accessed, what might be included and key points to consider. Finally, some other communication methods will be mentioned.

Motivations – why disseminate?

Why disseminate?

You may have spent many hours over several years, researching your area of interest, and through it you may have established new information to influence the actions and practice of others. Disseminating your research findings is therefore as important as carrying it out, especially if through it you have found information that could alter clinical activity, theoretical thinking or research in the future.

Dissemination of research findings is often seen as a final chore and sometimes omitted altogether. But not disseminating the findings of research should be seen as unethical practice. It is not ethical to consume all those resources (even if it is just your time) and collect all that data from willing participants if no-one learns from your experiences. Even negative results are important, if only to prevent others from unnecessarily repeating what you have done. Increasingly, research funding will only be granted if the research proposal has a robust strategy for widely disseminating the results of the study.

In addition to these reasons for disseminating your results, you may also have personal motivations for wanting to publicise your research. If you are a lecturer you may be expected to write papers and present at conferences in order to contribute to your university's research reputation, which may include participation in the Research Assessment Exercise (www.rae.ac.uk). If you are involved with the training of staff, presenting research may also be part of your job remit. If you have done your research as part of an educational course your supervisor will be encouraging you to publish and present it somewhere with their support.

There are many different ways of communicating research findings and all have validity but you must balance the impact your method will have and the number of people you will reach against the effort you may be putting in. You will talk about your research to your friends and colleagues but this will only inform a few who may be converts anyway. Your research may have produced findings which deserve wider publicity to enable changes in practice to be put in place.

Writing for publication

Writing for publication

'Now just listen to this one, will you,' he said 'and tell me whether it is good grammar and proper language.' [1]

The areas which you must consider for successful communication include: why you would wish to write an article for publication; when the best time to write an article is; and what sort of work you can write about. The final decision is where you can publish your work. There are many books devoted to the development of writing skills, but Graswell's *Writing for Academic Success* [2] deals very effectively with most of the areas I will describe.

Sooner or later, many people feel that they would like to share their ideas on paper with others. This often causes a problem known as writer's block. You sit in front of the computer and nothing comes out of your fingers onto the keyboard. It may be a relief to hear that writer's block happened regularly to a comic hero, Ronnie Barker. Ronnie wrote many a magnificent sketch but said writing was a skill he found difficult. So if writer's block happens to you then you can take some comfort from knowing that it has probably happened to most of us.

Successful writers and researchers are not the ones who have never encountered this phenomenon but the ones who have learnt how to deal with it successfully. It is important to remember when writing a journal article that you are not writing in order to win the Nobel prize for literature but just trying to convey your thoughts and organise your findings on a topic.

Why write for publication?

Why write for publication?

Writing for publication will often help you develop as a person and may aid the development of your career. For example, writing for publication certainly helps clarify your thoughts. It is useful to write articles based on the material that you are currently researching. Revisiting ideas and theories during the writing process really helps develop your work. Feedback from other people helps enrich your perspective on the research, and boosts your confidence and self-esteem.

However, you may find your own thoughts creating some obstacles to writing. Examples of these are provided by Day [3]:

'I can't write.'

'They will dismiss my ideas outright.'

'People will steal my ideas.'

'I am far too busy.'

Let us consider these obstacles in more detail. 'I can't write' is a common feeling amongst many of us. Journal articles may appear to be very well written – little wonder when some have been drafted and redrafted and commented on about five times. Do not be put off by this, as you will certainly find yourself redrafting articles based on comments and criticisms from your peers. Writing is a skill, and, like most skills, it becomes easier with practice.

Having your ideas dismissed may give you a feeling of despair or sometimes anger. But there may be good reasons for their dismissal. For example, you may have selected the wrong journal to publish your work in, or your ideas may need further clarification.

Experienced authors will often have an article rejected by one journal but accepted by another. This is the time to talk to experienced colleagues who have published articles, to get their advice on the best place to publish your work.

Having ideas stolen is a common fear. Perhaps you need to consider when to publish so that you are already viewed as the key player in your field, or present the results at a conference first to establish your ownership of the work. Finally there is the 'I am far too busy' reason and, whilst writing this chapter today, I most certainly am! This is not the place to go into detail on issues of time management, but is this really a valid excuse for wasting all the time that you have spent on the research project?

When is the best time to write?

When to write?

The answer to this differs according to what you are trying to publish. If you are trying to publish work from your thesis, then it may be better to wait until it is completed and you have asked your supervisors for their opinion. There is divided opinion as to whether PhD students ought to publish work before it is examined and, sometimes, the advantages of proving originality and contribution to the field of knowledge gained by publishing in a reputable peer-reviewed journal may be offset by the need to devote all available time to writing the work in a thesis format, or by issues of confidentiality or commercial sensitivity. However, for some research degree students this is seen as a part of the process and can be a part of the final award. It is best to check this with your supervisor before you start writing.

You may wish to adopt an incremental publishing strategy. You could initially present your work internally, perhaps as part of an institutional series of lunchtime meetings or similar professional development activity, where you can discuss your work in a friendly environment. Following this initial presentation of your work, you may wish to take the route of seminar, conference paper and then journal article. In this way you can gradually build up your confidence.

Another strategy you may wish to adopt is to co-author a paper with someone who has a good record of publication and can help you write and redraft articles. Most journals require all co-authors to have contributed to the research process, so this needs to be considered at the outset, as does the order of authors' names on the finished work.

What work is publishable?

What work is publishable?

This can be broken down into three main types of material:

- empirically based
- literature-based
- experience-based.

Empirically based research is often the easiest to get published. This may be because more journals are targeted towards dissemination of original research and there may be a perception that secondary research is not as important. However, with the growth of evidence-based practice, the secondary synthesis of research results is recognised as being important in its own right.

Additionally, rigorous methods for conducting systematic literature reviews and meta-analyses have addressed concerns about the quality of this form of research. Work that is based on experience can either be in the form of opinion pieces or the report of individual clinical case studies. Depending on the nature of the content, professional journals (rather than the academic, research-based ones) may be more appropriate vehicles for this sort of paper.

Where can you get your work published?

Where to publish?

When considering publication you need to target your journal carefully as each journal will favour particular types of material. It is best to seek advice about which journals in your field are most appropriate for these three types of material and the scope of the topics that they cover. In addition to the type of work which you wish to publish (see above) you may also wish to consider:

- the message you wish to convey
- personal objectives
- your audience and impact.

A guide to research for podiatrists

If you have interesting findings from your research, then you may feel you want to go for the most prestigious journal possible. However, you need to remember that these journals have an extremely high rejection rate. Perhaps in the early stages of your journey in publishing you need to consider a journal that may be more sympathetic to your requirements. Again, ask colleagues or supervisors about this and approach individual journals for their guidelines for publication. These can often be found on a journal's website.

You also need to consider your personal and professional objectives. You may be considering publication primarily as a mechanism for career progression or because you wish to contribute to the development of patient care within a service. You may want to use publication to trigger networking opportunities and further research opportunities. There is often a tension between research reputation and practice development. Publishing in journals with a high academic reputation will enhance the author's research reputation and provide evidence of this for future grant applications and your university's Research Assessment Exercise. However, these journals tend not to be those that are regularly read by practising clinicians, and the greatest clinical impact can often be gained by publishing in professional journals, such as *Podiatry Now*.

Your writing style will need to reflect your audience. Traditional research papers in academic journals tend to use a conventional scientific style. This usually involves writing in the third person, using passive verb forms (for example, 'the data was collected' rather than 'we collected the data'). Some journals which specialise in qualitative research may accept a more reflexive style, using the first person. Professional journals often adopt a more informal style of writing. The content of the paper needs be considered as well as the style. There is little point in writing a paper aimed at experts in the field, which may use specialised terminology and would assume a level of knowledge of the underlying concepts and theories, and submitting it to a journal with a general readership.

Audio-visual presentation

Audio-visual presentation

Journal articles will be read by subscribers and motivated, interested parties but it is said that people remember:

- 10 per cent of what they read
- 20 per cent of what they hear
- 30 per cent of what they see
- but 70 per cent of what they see and hear.

A presentation is therefore an efficient method of communication in terms of the ratio of effort to effect.

Why present?

Audio-visual presentation is usually an adjunct to a written article and so presenting is part of the process of disseminating the vital information that your research contains. Initially you might be put off by having to give a major presentation, unless you are well-practised in these skills from another role. But a presentation can be a good way of informing many people of your findings in a quick and engaging way.

When might you present?

The timing of your first presentation might be beyond your control. For instance, you may be faced with an opportunity to present to the largest and most appropriate audience you could wish for but feel ill equipped to deal with the situation. It is true that presentations require practice and skill to deliver well. For this reason you might enlist your supervisor's support and do it as a joint process or seek support from your NHS R&D research coordinator. If possible, take the opportunities that will best suit your dissemination needs and time commitments. Staff meetings, local groups and specialist groups will usually offer a more comfortable start as you will know many of the people and they are likely to be be sympathetic towards you. With practice, presenting will become easier.

What might you include?

You will need to think of your presentation much like a story containing a beginning, a middle and an end. The introduction should be a short summary of what you are there to do and the research you are presenting. The content will include obvious elements such as an outline of the aims, the methods used, the results and conclusions, with an outline of the consequences as you see them.

The clinical implications of your work will be particularly important. You will also need to identify further research or actions that could be taken as a result and it is often good to mention sources of support. Include some element that is light-hearted but appropriate to your research that can act as a memorable point to help people recall your presentation.

Get a friend to review it for obvious mistakes before you let everyone know that you can't spell. It is very important to have a practice run-through. The timing of your presentation will need to be accurate and you will need to speak more slowly than you usually do.

Which forums could you use?

The forum you choose may be dictated by circumstances, timing or opportunity. Some forums are easier to cope with than others. For example, staff meetings or local branch meetings are usually more comfortable places to present for the first time. They are populated by friends and acquaintances who will be supportive. They can be useful places to practise your presentation skills, delivery and content before going on to bigger venues. You are also more likely to get an honest response about your presentation as a whole, not just the content. These opportunities may be small in number but can, if you get asked elsewhere, add up to a significant number of people hearing your message.

If you have researched in your interest area, you are likely to be a member of that Special Interest Group and could use that, or a regional innovations or research and development event, as your next event. If you are a member of a specialist group, ask the secretary, contact your local NHS R&D coordinator for advice on whom to contact or speak to your supervisor for contact names that you can try.

Specialist groups will give access to like-minded people who understand the language of, and background to, the research that you are presenting. This can be both an advantage and a disadvantage. The language you use in your presentation can be more complex but you may get more probing questions about the detail of your research. However this should be easy for you to counter as you have lived with this research for a considerable time and can probably predict what the questions will be anyway.

Should you be presenting to a more mixed audience you will need to use less technically complex language. These events will test your delivery skills and ability to keep an audience interested in a subject of which they have no previous knowledge. In these instances, you will get questions on the techniques of analysis, practical questions or implementation issues. You are unlikely to have many specialists from your field to challenge the bulk of the content.

The ultimate presentation challenge is the national or international conference. Here you have a great opportunity to reach many people but presenting to a large audience can be daunting. This need not always be the case, as many conference attendees are inhibited when it comes to asking questions. It is true, however, that you need to make a good job of your presentation to keep a larger number of delegates interested in your subject. There are not many opportunities to present at national and international level but the obvious place to start is the Society of Chiropodists and Podiatrists Conference or similar. Usually you need to keep your eyes open for conference notifications and calls for papers. Your supervisor or NHS R&D coordinator may have knowledge of such events coming up and how to apply.

What things should you consider?

Your presentation may need to fill anything from a 10-minute slot to an hour. There are various important things that you must do to present yourself, and the research you have carried out, well. Some have been alluded to already but the best advice is to be well prepared. Check the time that you have to present in, make sure that you keep to it, and make sure what you say is relevant. A rule of thumb is to keep audio-visual aids simple – not too many slides and none of them over-complex in animation, colour or content. They can distract from what you are trying to say and may not work on the computer you have to use on the day. Practise your presentation delivery to make sure that your timing and emphasis are correct.

Ensure that you arrive early to download the presentation to the system you may be presented with, or to establish that your equipment is set up and works. Be on time to present and be familiar with the order and content of slides. Be familiar with your presentation equipment and the software that you are using, and ensure that you are using a compatible version. Have a contingency plan in case the presentation equipment fails either partially or completely. The content and style of your presentation needs to be appropriate and also stimulating and, above all, engaging for your audience.

Use notes if it will help but it is better to know your material well and present it with feeling and conviction. This is easier to do if you are not looking at notes. Most of all, look as if you are enjoying telling people about what you have discovered. If you are excited by it, they will be too.

Other methods of dissemination

Other methods of dissemination

Other means of communicating your message could also be available at regional, national or international events. The most common form is a poster presentation. This is an opportunity to present your research on a board of given dimensions (typically about A0). This needs careful planning as only the most important points can be displayed. You need to make sure that the text is large enough to be read at a distance of at least a metre away and it should be visually interesting, with appropriate pictures and graphs and so on. You will be expected to stand by your poster at fixed times throughout the conference to answer people's questions. Occasionally you will also be expected to make a 5-minute or even 15-minute presentation about your poster as well.

Finally

Writing up your research for publication or presenting your work may seem like a frightening propect at first but it is an essential part of the research process and brings tangible rewards for both you and your profession.

References

[1] P. O'Brian. *Master and Commander* (London: WW Norton and Company, 1990).

[2] G. Graswell. *Writing for Academic Success* (London: Sage, 2005).

[3] A. Day. *How to Get Research Published in Journals* (Aldershot: Gower, 1996).

Chapter 12
Closing the loop – putting research findings into practice
Wesley Vernon

If you wish to put your research findings into practice, the role of the manager is paramount. In NHS and non-single-handed practice situations, this would be a service or department or practice manager, or the senior partner in a private practice. In a single-handed practice, the podiatrist could be considered to have a personal clinical management responsibility and, in this sense, would be responsible for self-management.

For the podiatrist-manager, a range of tools are available to assist in implementing changes. These start with the general raising of awareness in the practice or service concerned, through memoranda, journal clubs, in-house newsletter articles and the like. Clinical supervision and mentoring also have powerful roles to play in such awareness-raising.

When considering evidence-based practice and practice development, your first task is to determine whether or not current practice is evidence-based. At this stage the skills covered in this book, associated with research-awareness and research-sensitivity, are required. An informed literature search into the relevant area of practice will determine the evidence available and a careful critique will help you determine the quality of the research and, by association, the amount of consideration that should be given to the findings of each paper. Consideration of the available literature in this way will provide a good indication of best practice in the selected area.

An appraisal of current local practice should then be undertaken, either through self-evaluation, monitoring, audit or by peer review, using conclusions from the literature reviewed to set the standards against which practice will be judged. After assessment, and through the resultant feedback, you should be aware of the necessary changes. These results can then be used to inform any changes in practice.

The management of change

Management of change

Sometimes, extensive changes may be needed, in which case you will need to consider the training needs of the individual practitioner concerned – either generic continuing professional development (CPD) requirements, or training focused on the practitioner's individual needs. In other cases, the changes required will be minor and will only require slight adjustments to current practice. In both situations, further monitoring and follow-up are required to check that the desired changes have been achieved.

A wide range of other managerial tools are available to drive change forward. These include incentive-based initiatives and reward for high performance, on the one hand, through to disciplinary and capability procedures where practice falls considerably short of acceptable and effective standards. Within the NHS, the Knowledge and Skills Framework [1], linked through the individual performance appraisal process to Agenda for Change [2], has a vital role to play. Agenda for Change has defined new pay scales for all NHS staff with certain gateways being linked to progression through these scales. The intention is to encourage staff to improve continuously in their practice in order to progress through these gateways and this process can be used to develop evidence-based practice approaches. While these initiatives are entirely NHS-based, similar approaches could be adopted in private practice situations.

Dealing with limited or no evidence

Lack of evidence

This discussion has so far assumed that there is an adequate amount of strong evidence upon which to base practice and the improvement of practice. It is not, however, uncommon to find that there is limited, low-quality or even a complete absence of evidence in an area of practice under consideration. Where this is the case, you should consider whether the available evidence is adequate to support the continuation of a practice or whether that practice should cease in the absence of supportive evidence. The same managerial processes can be used to take forward any changes required to do this.

Alternatively, the area of practice may be extensive, or the reflecting practitioner may believe that, even without supportive evidence, there is widespread anecdotal feedback or strong enough intuitive belief to warrant further investigation. The podiatrist would then need to consider whether or not they are willing to undertake additional work themselves to produce more robust evidence to inform future practice. If they are able to do it themselves, then a known researcher in the field could be approached to enquire whether they would be willing to consider the issues in question. If the podiatrist has the research skills, time and interest, they may wish to investigate the area themselves.

Both approaches will take time, involving inevitable competition for research funds and the creation of a high-quality research study which will be time-consuming and drawn-out. Such large-scale studies may, however, not be required. Although large projects provide high-quality, robust findings on which to base practice, research can also be undertaken at a more local, individual level in order to generate evidence to inform practice. While this would not be recommended for dramatic practice changes, and those which involve relatively high degrees of risk to a patient, they do nevertheless have a place in the initiation of evidence-based change.

Such approaches are inevitably cyclical and would follow an action research process as described in Chapter 5. Here, the practitioner or small group of practitioners would consider an area of practice and, through small-scale use of a variety of research approaches both quantitative and qualitative, would undertake small projects to inform and change practice. The period of reflection which follows the implementation of such change is a vital stage of the process and will not only allow the practitioner to focus on the results of the change adopted, good or bad, but also to consider future changes suggested in light of the findings.

Summary

The introduction of research findings into practice involves a process of change, which will inevitably require managerial consideration, whether that of a professional manager or a lone podiatrist who is self-managing their clinical practice. Where there is a strong pre-existing evidence base, which is not being followed, the requirements of change will be obvious and may require additional training. Where a strong evidence base is not apparent, the clinician can lobby for supportive research, or, alternatively, could adopt an action research approach with critical reflection in order to generate a reasonably robust change process on a local basis alone.

References

[1] Department of Health. *The NHS Knowledge and Skills Framework (NHS KSF) and the Development Review Process* (London: DH, 2004).

[2] Department of Health. *Agenda for Change* (London: DH, 2003).

Index

Index